Godsigns

Health, Hope and Miracles,
My Journey to Recovery

Suzy Farbman

Read The Spirit Books

an imprint of
David Crumm Media, LLC
Canton, Michigan

For more information and further discussion, visit

http://www.GodsignsBook.com

Cover art and design by
Rick Nease
www.RickNeaseArt.com

Published By
Read The Spirit Books
an imprint of
David Crumm Media, LLC
42015 Ford Rd., Suite 234
Canton, Michigan, USA

For information about customized editions, bulk purchases
or permissions, contact David Crumm Media, LLC at info@
DavidCrummMedia.com

Contents

Dedication

DEDICATED TO THOSE who share, have shared, or will share a life-threatening struggle and to those who love them. To Burton, my medical champion; to David and Andy and their families; to the friends and devoted medical team—the many caregivers, official and unofficial, who helped me through. Especially to Dr. John Malone who, after saving many lives, lost his far too soon.

Introduction

MY BATTLE WITH cancer turned out to be not just a physical quest, but a spiritual one as well. I was grateful to work with healers on both fronts.

During my treatment, I became convinced the process was divinely inspired. I met people, heard messages and received guidance when I most needed it. Guidance so finely tuned and pertinent and sometimes so quirky that, to me, it could only have come from a higher power.

In sharing my story, I refer to God as a "He" for ease of reading. What I really mean is "He/She", the all-gender eternal force that created life and sustains it.

While I refer to many friends by first names, I include Patsy and John Ramseys' last name. They were unfairly vilified in the media for so long. This is my small way of helping to right the perception of the loving couple we knew.

May my story bring hope and insight to you and your loved ones with your own challenges. May it awaken you to the signs I believe we all receive when we are sufficiently tuned in. There is nothing like a life-threatening illness to tune you in.

Watch with glittering eyes the whole world around you, because the greatest secrets are always hidden in the most unlikely places. Those who don't believe in the magic will never find it!

—**Roald Dahl**

CHAPTER 1

Godsigns

The only way out is through.

—Robert Frost

THE SEA SMELLED of sadness. As we dodged broken bits of clam, scallop, whelk and conch shells, the damp sand made me sad. The whoosh of waves made me sad. The cries of seagulls made me sad. This was the last Florida sunset we'd see for a while.

Ahead I noticed four women. They sat on a blanket, sipping drinks, chatting, laughing. It was March 2005. On the west coast, sunsets invite an extended cocktail hour. This group was enjoying the show. As we passed, I watched them, glad I had worn sunglasses so as not to seem rude. I envied their carefree ease, the fun they were having. I wondered who they were, where they came from. We passed them and kept walking. As the sun dipped closer to the blue horizon, Burton and I turned back toward our rented beach house on Longboat Key. The foursome remained where they were, still chatting and laughing.

On an impulse, I said, "I'm going to talk to them."

Burton frowned. "They look like they're enjoying their privacy."

I would not normally barge up to strangers on a beach. Especially when they seem to be having a good time without me.

Especially when wearing a frayed old jacket, no make-up and a chemo cap. Most especially when my husband discourages me. But occasionally I become stubborn. And cancer gets rid of inhibitions.

"They'll want to talk to me," I said. I let go of my husband's hand, climbed over a mound of drier, softer sand and strode up to the foursome.

"Where are we going for dinner?" I asked, pleased to have come up with a clever opener when cleverness had forsaken me in recent months.

"Right there," one said. She pointed to the high-rise apartment building behind them. "Nobody wants to be a designated driver."

Another lifted a bottle of champagne from a hole in the sand. "Join us," she said. "We have an extra glass."

I smiled, happy to be invited. I am happy to be invited most places. I like feeling included. But I shook my head. "Thanks anyway. What's the occasion?"

They were celebrating, they said. They had all turned fifty. They came from Wilton, Connecticut, had attended high school together and had been best friends ever since.

"Enjoy it," I said. Then, as if I hadn't sufficiently trodden on their cocktail gaiety, I added, "You don't know how much time you have. I turned sixty this year and came down with cancer." I patted my grey cotton cap.

They did not roll their eyes in a get-this-woman-out-of-here manner. They actually nodded and murmured sympathetically. One of them, with light blue eyes and no make-up, gazed at me with particular understanding. She pressed her hands to the navy sweatshirt over her chest. In a quiet voice, she said, "Fourteen years ago, I had cervical cancer. After I finished chemo, every day I'd ask my husband, 'Can I go without my hat yet?' He'd say, 'Not today, dear.' The four of us live in different parts of the country. We hadn't been together for ages. After I got sick, we realized we missed each other. That's when we started getting together. Now we do it every year."

She had short, streaked brown hair—about the color of mine, when I had it. Her cheeks were pink. She looked as healthy as a teenager. Before I had cancer, I had pretty much considered the disease a death sentence. Now each encounter I had with a real, honest-to-goodness survivor gave me hope.

The past three weeks had sped by. Three weeks without doctors or hospitals or toxic chemicals or burned flesh. We were scheduled to fly home to Michigan the next day. I had survived six months of treatment for stage-four uterine cancer. I faced one more hurdle. I needed another needle biopsy of my thyroid. If the tumor remained, I would require more surgery and radiation. Radiation had fried my vagina. I dreaded what it might do to my throat. As our freedom in Florida wound to a close, so did my spirits—up to that moment.

A wave of encouragement rolled through me. "Fourteen years," I said. "Good for you. I need to give you a hug."

She jumped up and wrapped her arms around me. I felt the press of her hands on my back, her chest against mine for three or four seconds, about as long as seemed appropriate for physical contact with a stranger on a beach.

Burton waited by the water. I rejoined him and took his arm. We resumed walking toward home, though I fairly floated.

I said, "I never even learned her name."

Early that evening, Burton dropped me off at the China Pavillion. (As a seventh-grade spelling bee champion, I abhor misspelled words, but it was their sign, and that was how it read.) Diners occupied almost every table of the small restaurant in Sarasota's St. Armand's Circle. The one free table was a drafty two-top near the door. Normally, with the outside temperature hovering in the low sixties, I'd have waited for another table or sought somewhere else to eat. Burton likes elbow room and dislikes two-tops. But we were running late for the theater; we liked the food here; and I knew we'd be served fast. I slipped on the sweater tied around my waist—I'm always prepared with an extra layer—and sat down.

At the table next to ours, an older couple was finishing their dinners. He had thin, white hair and wore a large hearing aid; she had a broad nose with deep pores. A clear plastic cane leaned against the wall behind her.

Still feeling sociable, I asked what they had eaten. Egg rolls and chicken chow mein, they said. Delicious, they agreed. Burton joined me. I ordered our usual: hot and sour soup for each of us and moo shu chicken to share.

I continued to buzz with the unexpected gift of my beach encounter. Within minutes, as we chatted with our fellow diners, I was rewarded again. The people beside us were Albert and Ida. They owned an apartment a few steps from our rented beach house. They had raised their children in Huntington Woods, Michigan, as we had. Albert had been a pilot in World War II. My father's name was Albert; he was a navigator in World War II. Their youngest daughter, Suzy, spelled the same, also has two sons. She suffered cancer in her mid-forties. And She Survived.

At some point in the conversation, we must have eaten our dinners. Burton must have rolled his helping into the flat cakes that came with the moo shu chicken. I must have combined mine with steamed brown rice. We both must have added hoisin sauce the way we always do. As much as I love to eat, I was too caught up in our conversation to pay attention to what I was chewing.

Burton is very polite. Usually he lets me choose my fortune cookie and takes the other one. This time he picked first. I opened the cellophane of the remaining cookie expecting something special, the way I'd bite into a truffle. I broke the cookie in half and unfolded the little white slip of paper. I caught my breath. *You will maintain good health and enjoy life.*

Burton and I had dined at the China Pavillion dozens of times. Albert and Ida had lived on Longboat Key longer than we had. They had never been there before.

Heading for the Florida Studio Theater in downtown Sarasota, I felt elated from my earlier encounters. We had tickets that night for *Metamorphosis*. Second row. Our subscription seats. This small theater had squeaky, hard chairs squeezed into narrow aisles and often ran out of bottled water. But they mounted intelligent productions with talented actors, and displayed posters with background on the theme of the play, and during intermission you could stand outside in balmy air.

I was surprised to see that a shallow pool of water took up most of the stage. Towels were draped over the backs of chairs in the first two rows. With my former curling-ironed and sprayed actual hair, or with Gertrude (my real-hair wig) aloft, I might have worried about being splashed. But that night I was wearing Frenchie, my synthetic wig. No problem.

The lights dimmed. The play held me captive.

Metamorphosis is a modern interpretation of ancient mythology, a subject I'd studied in high school but mostly forgotten. The water on stage symbolizes a swimming pool, a mirror, an ocean, a river, depending on the myth depicted. Near the end, Orpheus travels to the underworld, to the River Styx, to plead for the return of Eurydice, his late wife. Hades takes pity on him. Hermes may escort Eurydice out, Hades says, with one condition. He warns Orpheus not to turn around, to trust that Eurydice will follow. Orpheus marches straight ahead, resolute, looking forward. At the last second—he's out, she isn't—he glances behind. Eurydice falls back, leaving him forever.

I normally wait for someone else to initiate a standing ovation. That night, tears streaming down my face, I jumped up from my seat and applauded until my arms ached. The play beamed a message straight into my soul. I, too, had to keep forging ahead. No matter how hard the journey, I couldn't waiver as Orpheus had. I, too, had to trust, to march on without knowing the outcome. To believe in the possibility of recovery and in my doctors. And in the agonizingly long medical process into which dark river I would again wade the next day.

Burton and I drove back across the Ringling Causeway, the lights of Bird Key and Longboat Key twinkling ahead. Stars in the velvet sky rose and fell as we ascended and descended the new bridge. In our previous years of vacationing in Sarasota, a drawbridge lifted to let large boats pass underneath, causing frequent traffic backups. Now a permanent replacement curved over the bay. Underneath, graceful arches danced reflections in the water. Like the nearby tall sculpture, Unconditional Surrender, a sailor kissing a nurse, inspired by a famous *Life* magazine photograph marking the end of World War II, the bridge had become a Sarasota landmark.

My skin tingled. I felt as buoyant as the boats bobbing in the water below. I thought about how fearful I'd been earlier and about the events that had come together in the past few hours to lighten my attitude. The survivor on the beach. Albert, Ida and their daughter Suzy. My fortune cookie. Orpheus' challenge.

A thought popped into my brain, a thought so improbable that I pushed it back under the neat, tucked-in covers in my head. It poked its way out again. Ridiculous, I told myself, pushing it down once more. Crazy. But, like a little stuffed teddy bear, it peeked back out. I saw the tip of its ears, the furry crown of its head, its tiny glass eyes. The thought had a name. Godsigns.

Godsigns. The things that happened earlier. Things that had been happening since I became sick. Meetings. Casual remarks. Odd discoveries. They were signs from some benevolent force that either wanted me well or wanted me to know that all would be well, no matter the outcome. In a leap of faith higher than the stars above, I sensed these were signs meant for me. They were so delicately timed and orchestrated that—impossible as it seemed—they must have come from a mysterious, unknowable source. A source with infinite power, goodness and imagination. Pieces had been put in place and moved so perfectly that they could only have been masterminded by a chess player far more advanced than Bobby Fischer. By the ultimate chess player of the universe.

On one hand, it seemed the height of chutzpah to assume that people and events and conversations could have been arranged just for me. Who was I? Hardly someone who'd racked up points with the Almighty. I'd come to God in my fifties, but for selfish reasons. Because I had nowhere else to turn. Because prayer consoled me, helped me through worries about my mother and then about my marriage and now about my health. I was a nice person, a caring friend, a devoted parent and wife. But no Mother Teresa.

On the other hand, why not me? Why not any of us? I'd be a fool to dismiss the extraordinary turns that had occurred, especially in recent weeks. So many gifts had shown up in my life. It would be ungrateful not to appreciate them. I couldn't ignore the possibility that certain events were somehow designed to reassure me, to boost me up, to give me hope. Wishful thinking? Maybe. Illogical? You bet. But divine intervention is not a matter of logic. At least logic as far as we human beings can see. And even if these occurrences weren't specifically designed for me, they happened. That was magic enough.

No matter how loving my family and friends, or how encouraging my doctors, despite the degree to which medical technology had advanced, when I was in that small, sterile room taking CT scans, I was on my own. Me and my doubts. Each of us finds comfort in different ways. When we discover something that sustains us, I say chill the champagne, light the candles and embrace it. Believing the universe was on my side could help me to feel less alone. However magical the thinking, trusting in Godsigns just might help me to feel less afraid.

I had come to a yellow wood. I could take the intellectual path, a road of cynical disregard. I could give in to skepticism, toss these experiences aside as random or meaningless or trifling. Or I could treasure them, roll them around in my head and my heart as I would wiggle my tongue to savor a sip of a good cabernet. I could value their significance and welcome the grace they brought.

We turned on to St. Armand's Circle. Anticipating our return to the still-wintery Midwest, Burton had put the top down on the Corvette and turned up the heater full blast. The heater warmed our bottom halves; the night air cooled our cheeks. On the Avenue of Presidents, we drove past the Columbia, with its famous 1905 salad that my sister insisted on having whenever she visited from Santa Barbara and in which I was a willing partner. A few hardy diners sat outside. Tourists strolled the sidewalks, licking ice cream cones, checking out shop windows filled with t-shirts and bronze dolphins and multi-colored glass sculptures and dresses in pinks and greens.

"Godsigns," I murmured.

"What's that?" Burton often asked me to repeat myself. He had problems with his hearing, possibly from flying airplanes and shooting guns without adequate protection in younger years.

I wasn't sure I believed what I had said, but I repeated it anyway, in a firmer voice. "Godsigns. The things that happened today. I think they're signs from God."

Burton knew how much I dreaded going home. How much I dreaded facing the next day, the next month. He knew how much a spiritual connection had helped me through the preceding ones.

"I like the way you're thinking," he said.

Signs that kept me going had actually been occurring, and spurring me on, since the past summer when I was first diagnosed. They may well have been happening all my life, but it took getting sick to notice. That night in Florida I began to add them up, to wonder if something greater were involved. That night, our last in Florida for who knew how long, I began to wonder if they were more than lucky coincidences.

"Godsigns," Burton said. He cocked an eyebrow and looked at me. "Is there such a word?"

I shook my head. "I don't think so."

CHAPTER 2

It's Always Something

It's my job to sing from the wound.

—**Bonnie Raitt**

I LIMPED TO the red markers and teed up a ball. The first fairway stretched out before me, a par 4 expanse of emerald grass bordered by rough and trees. I thought about my key to the proper backswing, the acronym THE, the most common word in the English language. Turn, Hinge, Extend. "Don't think so much," Burton told me, but the golf swing came naturally to him. I drew back the club and cocked my wrists, straightened my left arm, began the down stroke. The instant I shifted my weight, pain shot through my left groin. A sharp, stabbing pain. Tears sprang to my eyes. My follow through collapsed. The ball skittered about fifty yards.

"Whoa," I said, wincing. "This isn't going to be my day."

Burton looked at me from the other golf cart and squinted. "We don't have to do this. We could drive back to Sarasota. See a doctor."

The sky was a wash of azure blue. The air smelled of jasmine. I didn't want to spoil anyone else's day. I have a tendency to put others first. It's a female thing.

I shook my head. "A little too much hay in last night's romp." I batted my eyes at him. "You guys play. I'll just putt."

It was March 2004, a year before the events that would spark my discovery of Godsigns. We had spent most of the past three months in a rented beach house on Longboat Key—pretty from the street, dilapidated inside, but featuring glorious sunsets that compensated for rusty screen doors and a saggy sofa. We were due to return home to Michigan in a week. If needed, I'd see my internist then. I sat in the cart, counting the months until summer. Thumb, index, middle finger. My injury should easily heal in three months. I'd be back on the golf course in June.

A few days before, Susie had called to invite us to Lemon Bay, their golf club near Boca Grande. I accepted gladly. The lessons I took the summer before up north, at the Rick Smith Academy where Phil Mickelson had trained, were paying off. I was shooting in the high 90s. As well as I had ever played. I was almost sixty. I walked or biked most days. Except for occasional flare ups of sciatica and some unpredictable stomach episodes, I was in decent shape. I had control of my life and my body. Or so I thought. My handicap was a semi-respectable 26. I looked forward to showing off my improved ability.

The morning of our golf date, I awoke feeling excited to see old friends and play someplace new. I swung my legs out of bed and stepped on the matted off-white carpet of our vacation rental home. The instant I put weight on my left side, the stabbing pain I later felt on the golf course first assaulted me.

The night before, Burton and I had gone on a date. Even couples married thirty-seven years needed time for romance. We had smelled the briny air as we walked across the Gulf of Mexico Drive to Pattigeorge's. We sat at the bar and shared miso-glazed sea bass. I drank a glass of house sauvignon blanc; Burton, a Foster's. We held hands and strolled back to our pink house, our king-sized bed. The evening progressed. I wrapped my legs around my husband and pressed a little harder than usual. A little too hard, I concluded the next morning when I stepped out of bed, felt a shooting pain and decided I had pulled a groin muscle. Strange things happened when you got older. Close up vision blurred. Wrinkles hung around. Now a rebellious groin.

I leaned back against the bed. For a change, Burton still lay there. Normally he was up reading emails or talking on the phone to our sons, also early risers, or driving to Publix for fresh bagels.

"Ow," I wailed. "My groin hurts. We must have overdone it last night. That's what a nice girl gets for confusing herself with Samantha."

Burton was beside me in an instant. He wore striped pajama bottoms and a Laurel Oak golf shirt. Laurel Oak was the golf club we joined when we first began renting on Longboat Key in Sarasota. Each year my husband bought several new, cotton golf shirts with the LOGC logo, believing members needed to support the pro shop. He wore them on the course and in bed. The sage-colored shirt he had on brought out his hazel eyes. His silver hair was still mussed from the pillow.

"Where does it hurt?"

I touched the junction between my crotch and my left thigh. Burton probed gently with his fingers. "I don't feel anything. Do you want to cancel golf?"

"I just pulled a muscle, I said. "Play over pain." It was the motto of our son's little league coach twenty-five-plus years before.

Days later, we flew back to Detroit. My *Sex in the City* injury still bothered me. I didn't think much about it, deemed it a temporary inconvenience. I thought I knew my body. I exercised—did mini push-ups, tummy tucks, walked or rode a bike most days. I had read an article which discussed something called a set point. If you did enough aerobic exercise to raise your set point, your body would metabolize food better and you could eat more. Since I loved food, this seemed a reasonable arrangement. And because I had a herniated L4/5 disc, it helped keep sciatica at bay. I figured I was doing what my body needed.

Now, however, my groin opted out of the arrangement. Trying to continue my daily exercise, I felt a searing pain each time I lifted my left leg. I continued to do mini push-ups and crunches but gave up the leg lifts.

I called my internist, a friend for many years.

"Give it time," Dr. Moss said. "A professional athlete who breaks a bone can be back in six weeks. A pulled groin muscle can sideline him for a season."

If the pros could tough it out, so could I. And so I babied my left side, and, as April turned into May and tulips into daylilies, I tried to overlook the pain. Besides, I had more important things to think about. *Back from Betrayal*, my first book, was published in early May, soon after our return from Florida. It was a memoir about how my husband and I survived a marriage crisis. The book revealed how my husband's affair almost destroyed our marriage. And how hard work, confronting the truth, and becoming more tuned in to each other slowly brought us back together. Writing about our experience was therapy for me. The book told the story of our gradual journey to forgiveness and understanding. I considered it a love story. Burton had written the afterword. Our family had been featured on *Oprah*. A planned two-segment appearance turned into five segments and a second show as well. Both aired twice. I had received, and answered, emails from hundreds of readers. I was busy calling magazines, doing radio interviews, giving readings, checking ratings. Too busy to worry about a minor sex injury.

I've been busy all of my life. Before Burton and I had children, I worked full time. Burton was getting started in real estate, and I was proud that we survived on my salary, $110 a week. We lived in a small duplex in Detroit's Palmer Park neighborhood. We washed dishes by hand. One stifling summer we scraped together enough money to buy an air conditioner for the master bedroom. I took the bus to work. Despite the financial strain, those were happy times. We were both developing exciting careers—I, in journalism; Burton, in real estate.

I loved being a journalist—finding a hot story or interviewing newsmakers or, later, creating a striking fashion or design layout. I enjoyed being friendly with wives of auto execs, attending black-tie events with society and business leaders. I earned a front-page story in status trade publication *Women's Wear Daily* on the Detroit riots and a two-page center spread on glamorous Cristina Ford, then-wife of Henry Ford II. I broke the story of maverick auto designer DeLorean's facelift in a gossip column I wrote for the *Detroit News*. Later, as a regional design editor for *Better Homes and Gardens*, I gained national attention for Detroit designers and architects. As a journalist (part-time after our first son was born), a mother of two active boys and wife of a rising real estate executive, I was busy.

For most of my life, I was too busy to think much about religion, which had proven complicated and uncomfortable in my own family's history. My first memoir, which caught the attention of Oprah and her millions of viewers, did reveal how Burton and I turned to spiritual practices. Earlier in our marriage, I would not have expected the trials that befell us or that prayer would help to draw us back together. But it gave us the sense that something bigger was in charge. Prayer made the impossible possible.

Soon, as hard as I tried to ignore the pain in my groin, my anxiety would escalate into full-blown fear of the invisible entity growing within me. Though I didn't know it yet, I was entering a realm even bigger and more frightening than my earlier worries about my marriage. I would find myself in a circle of top medical professionals, using the world's most sophisticated scanners, who couldn't seem to agree on what alien force had invaded my body. That nagging pain in my groin would send me on a journey even more disorienting than repairing a broken relationship.

As a journalist, I was trained to look for the facts. But the facts of my case would prove so confusing that I needed to find comfort elsewhere. My life's work had prepared me to keep searching for truth and to grab hold when I found it. The truths I would find came from many sources. While I wouldn't name these insights Godsigns for quite a while, wisdom from friends and strangers, guidance from books and numbers, quirky coincidences would all provide spiritual support. My friends' religious traditions varied, but each carried a little light of inspiration. The sparks were there if I was watching. The wisdom was there if I was listening.

In the months ahead, I would watch and listen and learn. Like a good journalist, wiser from the surprising insights I had gleaned from our struggle to save our marriage, I opened my eyes and ears. I opened the pages of my journal. I opened my heart.

Toward the end of June 2004, Burton and I headed north to our farmhouse near Charlevoix, Michigan. I tried to play golf again. My regular partner, Lynne, now routinely hit past me. It still hurt to swing through. When my drive on the third hole of the Belvedere golf course landed in the creek instead of carrying about 100 yards, I stopped keeping score.

Several months before, a routine check-up showed my blood pressure had risen. Dr. Moss had prescribed medication and asked me to return in a few months to recheck my pressure. I had scheduled an appointment for mid-July, when I knew we'd be in town. Our younger son, Andy, and his wife, Amy, were expecting a baby, our first grandchild.

Back in Detroit, Dr. Moss approved of my blood pressure. Sitting on his examining table, I touched the left side of my crotch. "This still hurts," I said. "It's been four months."

He frowned, folded his arms. "Four months is a long time. Let's take an x-ray."

I stood before a machine, pressed my pelvis forward, heard a zap. Minutes later, my doctor sat behind his blonde wood desk, studying the x-ray of my hip.

"I don't see anything," he said. "Must be a groin pull. Be patient."

That night at Beaumont Hospital, where Andy was born, I discovered how much more humane labor had become. With both of my pregnancies, I suffered through eight hours of painful contractions. During active labor, Amy received an epidural which delivered a local anesthesia. I marveled at my daughter-in-law's ability to make pleasant conversation rather than groan and curse as I had at decreasing intervals, despite our Lamaze training. We chatted about what sex the baby would be (Burton and Amy: boy; Andy and I: girl) and discussed color schemes for the nursery. When the anesthesia was halted, Burton and I left for the waiting room. In about half an hour, a nurse came to get us. I speed-walked as fast as a sore groin would permit to the end of an eternally long hallway. Andy met us at the door to Amy's room, a big smile on his face.

"A healthy baby," he said, relishing the suspense.

"Boy or girl?" Burton prompted.

"Ten fingers. Ten toes."

"The baby's name?" I demanded.

"Alexis," he said, grinning as though he had just nailed a three-point long shot with a basketball. "She's a beauty."

Many of my friends couldn't wait to have grandchildren. I was too busy leading my life to think much about it. But the instant I entered the shiny, clean hospital room and beheld a tiny, pink infant, swathed in a blanket, lying in Amy's arms, I understood why normally rational people go daft about grandchildren. Amy offered the baby to me. Alexis—such a big name for such a little person—had navy blue eyes and dark, silky hair and minute hands that curled around my little finger. She smelled of strawberries and lavender. Before long, I thought, this perfect little miracle would be able to speak the name Gigi, the grandmother name I had decided I on. Before long, she would take her first steps. Before long, I would read to her *Eloise* and *Madeleine*, books I had loved.

Burton, always prepared with a camera, snapped several pictures of me holding Alexis' cheek next to mine. Part of us, I realized, would live on through this amazing new life. As I beamed for the camera, I felt all the more grateful that Burton and I had stayed together. Were here together. Could enjoy this moment together.

A week later, on Friday, the phone rang in our farmhouse. I was rinsing cherries from neighboring Friske's Farm Market. I dried my hands and picked up the receiver.

"I had a radiologist look at your x-ray," Dr. Moss said. "There's an abnormality in your pelvic bone. It looks like you have a small fracture. I want you to come home for an MRI."

"We'll be back in two weeks."

"I want you here sooner than that. I booked you an appointment for Monday."

"Aren't you the organized one."

I have a gift for not borrowing trouble. Some would call it denial. I didn't ask my doctor the reason for his sense of urgency. I'd try not to think about it until Monday.

Burton looked up from the salami he was slicing. "Who was that?"

"Gordon. He wants me home on Monday for an MRI."

"MRIs can be scary. Do you want me to come?"

I shook my head. I had already come up with a new diagnosis.

"Summer's too short already," I said. "I won't be afraid. I'll close my eyes and pray. Gordon will give me something for osteoporosis. I'll be back up north in a day."

After the MRI, I drove toward my office, wondering how bad my osteoporosis was. Within minutes, my cell phone rang.

"Come to my office in an hour," Dr. Moss said. "I want to talk to you."

I didn't call Burton. Why worry him when it wasn't necessary. Dr. Moss will prescribe a bone strengthener, I told myself. He'll warn me about sexual acrobatics at my age and send me on my way.

By the time I reached Dr. Moss' private corner office, I felt jittery. Relax, I scolded myself. Other women your age have osteoporosis. Look at Sally Field. Boniva helped her. Somewhere in my consciousness there hovered a question about what could be so serious that my doctor wanted to see me right away. I slapped my cheek as I do when I feel sleepy while driving and pushed that doubt out of my head. I focused instead on the photos of my doctor's wife and daughters displayed on a beige laminate credenza then jerked my gaze to the print behind his blonde wood desk.

Hanging on the wall was a Calder sketch for a large, red outdoor sculpture resembling a flamingo. It carried me back to my dating days with Burton. I was a fashion copywriter for Chicago-based Carson Pirie Scot department store, my first job after graduating from the University of Michigan. Burton ran the Chicago collections office of Detroit-based Advance Mortgage. At lunchtime, on sunny days we often walked to nearby Daley Plaza in the Loop. There was a new fifty-foot-high Picasso sculpture of Cor-Ten steel in front of a tall office building. Sitting on a low granite wall, munching sandwiches, we debated whether the veined head represented the face of a woman or a baboon. I liked knowing that my boyfriend, a street-smart guy who had been a poor student, showed an interest in art. Each time we visited that plaza, we noticed the same homeless man, wearing a dirty, torn brown sweater, sitting several yards away. Before we returned to work, we'd give him the rest of our sandwiches.

My doctor walked in, wearing a white coat, looking tanned and professional.

I gestured to the credenza. "I figure doctors display pictures of their pretty wives to discourage predatory patients," I said. "I approve."

Gordon is normally good humored. In this case, he sat down without smiling.

"Suzy," he said, looking at me. I couldn't read his expression, but it wasn't his usual easy-going face. I imagine most doctors become inured to giving bad news, but Gordon was a friend as well as my doctor. The conversation couldn't have been easy for him. I realize this in retrospect.

"It's my practice to send x-rays taken in this office to a radiologist. The radiologist who looked at your hip x-ray was concerned. He wanted you to take an MRI. I had him check it right away." He paused. "There are lesions in your pelvic bone."

"Lesions?" My voice rose. The air left my lungs. Denial exited my brain. I recognize a euphemism when I hear one.

"Could we be talking … about … cancer?"

His lips pressed together. He nodded. "We could."

That homeless man shuffled through my head. I saw the half-nod he gave us. I wondered if he appreciated our leftovers. Or resented them.

My heart pounded so hard I was sure my doctor could hear it.

"But you don't get tumors from sex," I whispered.

"I think an injury occurred because the bone was already compromised."

I must have said goodbye. I probably hugged him because that's what you do when you're upset. I probably even said thank you because that's how I was raised. Thank you? Thank you for what?

So much for control of my life and my body.

I staggered down the stairs and out into the warm air. I found my car, fumbled with the remote opener, sat in the car gasping for breath, trying to see the numbers on my cell phone through the blur.

"Hello?" Burton said.

"I need you here."

CHAPTER 3

The Broken Places

*The world breaks everyone and afterward
many are strong in the broken places.*

—Ernest Hemingway, *A Farewell to Arms*

BARIUM SULFATE CONTRAST dye tastes
better when refrigerated, the nurse said. Better than Drano, I
thought. Between sips of chilled, chalky liquid, I pressed half a
lime to my tongue. Every few swallows I still choked on the vis-
cous lemon-flavored sludge.

Alexis slept peacefully in her portable car seat. For the rest
of us, peace was more elusive. Andy, Amy and David, our older
son, sat in our library, trying to distract us. Andy talked about
baskets he had scored in his last weekly game with friends.
David, about his recent trip up north to prepare for bow hunting. They talked about the baby, business, travel plans. David
shared a joke he'd read on e-mail. I wondered if I'd ever find
anything funny again.

Later, in bed I eyed the pile of magazines on my night stand.
I liked being culturally savvy. I picked up knowledge about
matters as random as how to grill an artichoke (boil first; cut in
half; brush with olive oil; sprinkle with spicy seasoned salt) or
the recent scandal over Janet Jackson's nipple flash on national
TV (deliberate, I thought) or the launch of the then largest

passenger ship ever built, the Queen Mary 2 (three and a half times as long as Big Ben is tall). I opened *New York* magazine. Unable to concentrate on the latest sushi restaurant, I tossed *New York* on the sage-green wool carpet. I picked up *W* to check out the next season's fashions. Tropical prints and pearlized finishes. I may not have a next season to pearlize. *W* landed on top of *New York*.

Books of affirmations had helped me survive our marriage crisis. (I had developed the habit of calling our recent problems "our marriage crisis." It seemed a more delicate turn of phrase than "infidelity.") I pulled out Iyanla Vanzant's *One Day My Soul Just Opened Up* and reread words I had underlined five years before. "Most of the time, the thing we fear has absolutely no power, yet we brace ourselves for the worst possibility. You are not being tested. You are being fortified."

A Xanax and an Ambien further fortified me. Burton, who rarely took drugs to sleep, gulped an Ambien as well. Soon, he snored softly. Despite chemical support, I flipped back and forth in bed. My mind whirred.

Despite our problems, Burton was a good man with a good heart. But staying with a wife whose survival had slammed into question seemed a lot to ask of any husband, especially one whose wife had just shown the world his failings. My readers had shared stories about husbands who had bailed when they got sick. I was afraid to tell Burton about my worries, as though speaking them could make them come true. This tendency to avoid talking about concerns was one I should have gotten over. But old habits are as sticky as hair gel.

Burton was never a quitter. He built his career on making investments and staying with them. I had often kidded that he had a problem with his hearing. When someone said "no," he heard "yes." Still, I had never been really sick before. And although our relationship seemed renewed, I couldn't be sure it would hold. If Burton left me, I'd be dropped in the laps of my kids, who had lives of their own. The prospect of burdening my children with my neediness, as my mother had done to me, churned my gut.

Among mostly favorable reviews, a few hateful ones had shown up on Amazon.com. Someone claimed to know me, called me a phony and a social climber. I assumed the nasty reviews were generated by the ex-other woman I wrote about, or by readers unable or unwilling to reconcile in their own relationships. At least it comforted me to see them that way. I decided to stop checking on Amazon. I couldn't afford to take in negative energy. As important as my book had been for the last five years, I needed to let it go. It would take care of itself. Or not.

Worrying about my next day's CT scans, I picked up a new journal. Maybe the bone abnormality is congenital or isn't related to my ovaries, I wrote.

Green numbers on my clock glowed 2:30, 3:30, 4:30.

I stared out the car window at boarded up and burned out buildings, vacant lots littered with beer cans and plastic bags, storefront churches, wig shops and liquor stores shielded with metal fences. I smelled the odor of smoke. Four anxious days and three sleepless nights had dragged by since the word cancer was first aimed at me. Burton, David and I drove in silence to the Karmanos Cancer Institute, about five miles north of downtown Detroit. Our brother-in-law Neal, a retired orthopedist, came, too. Burton wanted to be sure we had someone objective, with medical expertise, on our team.

With falling auto sales, Detroit had suffered in recent decades. Burton and I had done what we could to fight the decline. We had served on boards and run charity events for our museum, our zoo and historical society. Burton had made several risky investments downtown and turned a profit on most of them.

To the west, the golden spire of the Fisher Building pierced the blue sky. When I became engaged to Burton and moved back to Detroit, I worked across the street in the building which had once housed Saks Fifth Avenue. Three decades later, our sons purchased the Fisher Building, filled most of its empty spaces and continued to run it. Burton and I loved watching David and Andy operate the real estate company we had started. When our sons bought and revived buildings in the city, we took special pride. As I wondered if I'd get to share many more of their accomplishments, I felt acid bite into the top of my stomach.

Near the hospital, banners hung from light poles: Early Detection Saves Lives. I still hoped I didn't have cancer. If I did, I prayed we were early enough.

In the busy lobby, we were met by a pert redhead, Lynn Sinclair, the assistant to the hospital director. She walked us to the gynecology department. Dr. John Malone was chairman of obstetrics and gynecology for the nearby Wayne State University School of Medicine, Lynn said. He was a nationally-respected expert in gynecological oncology, a term even harder to contemplate than it was to pronounce. She gazed at me with piercing blue eyes and promised, "You're in the best of hands."

I was stunned to be sitting in the lobby of a cancer center, waiting to meet a surgeon. I might as well have been visiting Mars. I had never been in a cancer hospital before, had hoped to live a long life without ever doing so. How naïve I had been. Several women sat nearby, some in scarves or caps, their faces pale and somber. Most were silent, though someone else sat with them. All of us, I realized, were glad for the company and grateful for the support, but in the end we were on our own.

What was I doing here? All along I'd taken steps to prevent my ever needing such a place. I ate low-fat meals and broccoli and blueberries full of antioxidants. I did not consume artificial sweeteners. I climbed stairs, got check-ups. We didn't live near power lines or in contaminated neighborhoods. But I did have radiation for acne as a teenager, had taken birth control pills as a young woman, used a Copper 7 intrauterine contraceptive device for several years. The last few years had been stressful. Could any of those causes have landed me here?

My heel jiggled as I glanced around the high-ceilinged reception area. I noticed artworks by several Detroit artists, some of which looked familiar. I had supported local artists since 1977 when I bought a piece by Michael Luchs in honor of our tenth anniversary. A collage resembling a rabbit, it was made of rags and fence wire on a jagged piece of plywood and hung in our stairwell at home. I felt like that rabbit—vulnerable, trapped, afraid.

The gadget beside to me buzzed. My heart thudded.

"Let's do it," Burton said.

Burton put his hand on the small of my back. He propelled me through a door into a bright corridor of examining rooms. Outside one of them, two names were penned on a white board: Farbman/Malone.

There must be a mistake, I decided. Dr. Malone will find it.

A small plaque was propped in a corner of the examining room: Cancer cannot cripple love; it cannot shatter hope. The message was meant to provide encouragement. It only reminded me of a fate I didn't want to consider.

Dr. John Malone strode in to the small room, badges dangling from the neck of his white jacket. His cheeks were pink, his hair almost as white as his coat. A sign of experience, I thought. He'll figure out what is really wrong.

"I've reviewed your tests," he said, looking at me. "What worries me is the bone. Cancer doesn't spread to the bone until it's late in the process."

Pressure mounted in my stomach. Take it easy, I told myself. He hasn't examined you.

Dr. Malone, Neal and David left the room. Burton stayed. I took off the pants to my yellow terrycloth jogging suit. As a fashion journalist earlier in my career, I believed clothes said something about their wearer, about her aspirations, how she wanted to be perceived. I chose yellow that morning. If I looked bright and healthy, I must be bright and healthy.

Dr. Malone knocked, walked back in, nurse Tina behind. As he slipped on rubber gloves, I placed my heels in hard stirrups. My knees trembled. A cold, metal speculum pressed into my vagina. Fingers probed, uncomfortable but not painful. I smelled Vaseline, closed my eyes, focused on breathing. Seconds later, the doctor snapped off his gloves and left me to dress.

David and Neal returned. So did Dr. Malone. I held my breath.

"I'm not sure what we're dealing with," he said. "I don't see any lesions, but I feel a large mass. Whatever it is, it needs to come out. I recommend a complete hysterectomy, as soon as possible. We'll open your stomach from your navel to your pubic bone and remove your ovaries and uterus. On your way out, stop by the lab for a blood draw. I want to run a CA 125 test for possible ovarian cancer."

The pressure in my gut intensified. My ovaries and uterus had produced two amazing babies and minded their business ever since. They had cooperated through annual check-ups, never giving me trouble, not even a miscarriage nor the painful menstrual cramps so many other girls suffered. I was grateful for their quiet, undemanding presence. Now I was being forced to give up part of me. My female organs were deemed disposable, apples that had rotted.

"Can you enter through my navel?" I asked, sounding more intelligent than I felt.

"Normally, yes. In this case, no. I need to view your abdomen for possible spread."

I swallowed hard, tried to dredge up my best professional interviewer voice. The words came out in a whisper. "What are the chances the mass is malignant?"

"Sixty/forty."

I started to shake.

On the way home in the car, Burton said, "I liked him. He's a real professional." I wailed, "He said there's a sixty percent chance I have cancer."

"Forty percent you don't. I'm focusing on that."

Home later, knowing something was seriously wrong, not knowing what, I felt panic clawing through my chest. My limbs twitched. I walked into the kitchen and picked up a pile of mail. Five tall windows spanned the back kitchen wall. The house stood at the edge of a ravine. In summer, we looked out at a green canopy of sugar maple leaves that yellowed and reddened in the fall. Smaller windows sat above the taller ones, a clerestory printed with the first line of my favorite Robert Frost poem. Two roads/diverged/in a/yellow/wood … The quote appeared sandblasted, but was done with frosted plastic letters. The type was simple, classic Times New Roman. My friend Mary Lou, an art director, laid it out for me. A sign man copied her drawing. I had written about design for much of my career and loved unique details. The windows were among my favorite details in the house. With sixty/forty thrumming in my head, I wondered what road we should take. Whether we'd find the right one. Whether there was a right one.

When Burton and I first married, in 1967, we could barely afford to dine out, no less pay for an entire house. We rented a small but affordable duplex in Detroit. Our olive-green sofa came from Burton's mom who also crocheted us a mustard and olive afghan. The neighborhood wasn't the safest. Palmer Park, across the street, had some shady characters lurking. I was a correspondent for Fairchild Publications, a group of respected national trade magazines. I wrote mostly about fashion and home furnishings retailing. I would go on to work for the *Detroit News* as a columnist and feature writer, then to free lance for several years, and then to work as a regional design editor for national magazines. We would no longer need the money I brought in. But the year we wed, Burton was just getting started in real estate. He depended on commissions, which were few. We had one car, Burton's old beige Plymouth Barracuda—u.b.u., as we say about certain golf shots, ugly but useful. On warm summer nights we'd put a pork roast on the rotisserie in our small back yard, take our golf clubs to the Palmer Park public course, play nine holes and return home to consume juicy, hot meat with applesauce. When Burton closed a real estate deal, we splurged on lobster and creamed spinach at Joe Muer's, a popular Detroit seafood restaurant, the original long since closed. Burton liked his lobster broiled. To save money, I shared my husband's. Not as moist as the steamed preparation I preferred, but still delicious, and flavored by Burton's most recent commission check. Marriage is made of concessions, some so small you scarcely know you're making them.

Trying to open a letter, I poked my thumb with the silver letter opener we had brought back from a trip to Egypt.

"Shit," I said, holding my thumb under cold running water.

"Let me look," Burton said. He turned my thumb back and forth in his hand. Burton had hands as soft as a baby's bottom. I slathered mine with lotion but they never felt as smooth as his.

"You're going to live." He kissed my thumb. "That should help."

Despite my insecurities, Burton had shown no sign of abandoning me in my delicate condition. He had not only stuck with me, he seemed more caring and tender than ever.

I took a centering breath. "I need a favor," I said. "The biggest favor I've ever asked. I'm afraid to get involved in the medical side of my case. I'd drive myself crazy thinking about everything that could go wrong. The most I can hope to do is shore myself up spiritually." I paused. I was about to ask a favor which would interrupt his sleep time, his TV time, his golf game, his peace of mind, though I guessed his peace of mind had already been interrupted.

"Will you take over?"

Burton's hazel eyes drilled into mine. "Consider it done."

"Bless you," I said, feeling relieved. Burton often lost focus in routine activities. He forever misplaced keys, glasses, papers, tickets, but laughed about it and eventually found them again. If I lost something, I panicked, which is why I carefully put keys in my purse, glasses in drawers, papers and tickets in files. But even with his disorganized ways, Burton was the best person I knew in a crisis.

Soon after, I answered the phone.

"This is Dr. Malone. Good news. Your CA 125 markers are low."

"Then I don't have ovarian cancer?"

"Probably not."

I blinked back tears.

Burton called Patsy Ramsey, a friend and cancer survivor. He put me on the phone.

"Buck up," she said. "Cancer isn't a death sentence anymore."

Ten years before, a new house was being built a block away from our summer home in Charlevoix. Then a regional design editor for *Better Homes and Gardens* and several special interest publications, I wandered around the construction site. The house had high ceilings, large windows overlooking the harbor below, a side porch and a Victorian feel. I hoped the home would turn into a subject for one of the magazines I represented.

After the family moved in, I knocked on the door. Patsy Ramsey invited me in. Short brown fuzz sprouted from her skull. She was thirty-six, recovering from stage-four ovarian cancer. "Hence, the do," she'd said, rubbing her head. She talked proudly about that morning's accomplishment. She and her daughter had decorated JonBenét's training-wheeled bike with red, white and blue bunting and streamers. Their creation won first prize in the town's annual bike-decorating contest. Together they had walked their award winner down Bridge Street in the Fourth of July parade. JonBenét, then three, scampered through the living room, holding a Cabbage Patch Doll. A year later, on another visit, I'd see JonBenét again. This time she had just won the Little Miss Charlevoix competition. Her blue, first-place banner was slung across her four-year-old frame.

In 1996, the Ramseys' decorating was complete. The couple worked with Linda Mason, a Charlevoix designer whose work I had featured before. The house was a natural for my magazines.

It included an upstairs dorm room with six twin beds covered in unmatched colorful quilts and a cloud-painted ceiling in JonBenét's bedroom. The downstairs was done in pretty pastel traditional furnishings. Outside, a real-wood white picket fence surrounded the white clapboard-sided residence. Patsy and John, who had become friends, agreed to let me propose their house for a design feature. That fall I took scouting slides inside and out, submitted a proposal to *Home Plan Ideas*, and received an unusually large assignment for about a dozen pictures. I decided to wait until the following summer to take the photos, ensuring blooming flowers outside and blue water and sailboats below.

Several weeks later, the day after Christmas, Burton and I sat at the breakfast table of our new home in Franklin, reading the newspaper. I always started with the lifestyle section; Burton, with the front. "No," he moaned. "I can't read this out loud." He passed me the article reporting JonBenét's murder. After losing her only daughter, Patsy stayed in bed and out of touch. I never completed my assignment. A year later, Patsy got up and back to living and to raising their son. JonBenét's murderer was never found. Patsy and John were wrongly suspected for several years and hounded by tabloids. Defending themselves and futilely seeking their daughter's killer destroyed John's business and their life savings. Remarkably, Patsy's cancer didn't return for another six years. In the last two, she had received chemo for two recurrences.

On the phone that afternoon, Patsy told me she had participated in early studies of the chemo drug Taxol, conducted at the National Institute for Health. She promised that today's drugs minimized the nausea she had suffered. If I had to undergo chemo, she advised me to have a catheter, or port, implanted in my chest during my hysterectomy. "It will save your veins," she said.

"If I do have cancer, I'm afraid to hear my chances of survival," I said.

"I didn't want to know mine either." Her voice was tinged with a lilt of West Virginia, where she was born. "I told my doctors: I'm no good with numbers. I'm not a statistic. I'm a child of God."

Several years later, she learned what her chances had been of surviving five years. Five percent.

Patsy was right, I decided. If I had cancer, which I still prayed I didn't, I wouldn't ask my chances either.

During treatment, Patsy found comfort in scriptures. "While they were pumping poison into my veins, there was one line I repeated over and over." As she told it to me, I wrote it in my journal:

In the shelter of his wings, I shall seek my refuge, until these calamities have passed. (Psalms 57)

I was too paralyzed by fear to realize it then. I would come to see that God spoke to me in many ways. Through riddles, coincidences, mysteries, dreams. Through people like Patsy. At the time, I was grateful for her counsel, but unaware of the bigger picture.

"Call if you need me," she said. "Any time. Day or night."

Dr. Michael Mott, an orthopedic surgeon, pressed my groin and rotated my legs.

"Any pain?" he asked.

"No," I said, hoping it was a good sign.

Five days had passed. Because my pelvic bone was involved, we had not proceeded with Dr. Malone's recommendation of an immediate hysterectomy. I lay on a table in the examining room of a bone specialist, accompanied by my same support team plus my girlfriend Brenda. Her husband, Howard, had hung out with Burton as teens. We had attended each others' weddings. But Brenda and I bonded over clothes.

After working as a fashion copywriter in Chicago, I returned to Detroit and became a reporter for *Women's Wear Daily*. Brenda was then the fashion coordinator for Saks Fifth Avenue in Detroit. (During college, I had worked for that store, for a branch in Ann Arbor, and also for the flagship store on Fifth Avenue in New York.) I had loved the Detroit store since I was a girl. The first floor featured glass cases filled with chiffon and silk scarves and leather gloves, sparkling brooches and cosmetics. It had a big millinery department and polished marble floors. It smelled of Shalimar and Arpege. My grandmother took me shopping there, in the pre-teen and junior departments on the second floor. She always bought me something wonderful—a gold circle pin or a plaid, pleated skirt or a cardigan sweater to button down the back. With our mutual love of fashion, when Brenda joined Saks, it seemed inevitable that we would become close.

As a journalist, I chronicled my friend's rising career and style opinions. Brenda, who never had children, traveled the world viewing couture shows, scoping out trends, designing products. There were moments when I was changing diapers or seeking babysitters (I once made twenty-seven calls before finding one) that I envied Brenda's glamorous life. She knew Armani and Versace and St. Laurent and wore their designs to their couture shows. I wore sweatsuits to pick up carpools.

After 9/11, Brenda began working for interfaith peace. In recent years she had spent countless hours meeting with Christians, Muslims and Jews, creating an interfaith teen play, installing Jewish libraries in mosques. Despite skepticism from many other Jews, Brenda built trusting friendships with moderate Muslims. She prided herself on having several imams on speed dial.

Brenda still loved fashion and often agreed to shop with me. Shopping is a unique female bonding ritual. Whoever makes you look better makes you feel better. When Burton and I skidded apart, Brenda helped prop me back up. She pushed me into sexier underwear and stretch jeans. We also golfed together. Six years before, she was the sole witness to my hole-in-one. When we saw that little, dimpled white orb sitting in the cup, Brenda shrieked and jumped up and down as excitedly as I did.

But that was then. I was no longer jumping up and down.

Dr. Mott left the room to review my x-rays. Burton sighed. David fidgeted with a string. Brenda put her arm around me. When you're in a doctor's office waiting to hear a diagnosis, your breath, your heart, the seconds ticking by hang suspended.

Dr. Mott returned and reeled off some technical terms. I had a lytic lesion of the right ischial pubic rami junction. I also had a lesion of the superior pubic rami on the left. I wrote as he spoke, for something rational to think about later, when my brain might again start to function.

"These lesions could be anything. They might not be malignant." My heart lifted. "I suspect they are." And fell again. "They appear aggressive. This looks like metastatic carcinoma to the pubic bones. Bone cancer comes from someplace else. In women, most often from the lung, breast, kidney or thyroid. Your bone lesions might not relate to the mass in your uterus but probably do."

Dr. Mott had scheduled me for a CT guided core-needle biopsy. Our little group traipsed through the modern hospital into an adjoining older one. We rode a dreary elevator to a dreary basement hall. Burton held my arm tight, as though he could will his strength into me. My feet moved on their own, zombie-like. I had slipped into some grim alternate reality.

In Interventional Radiology, we were greeted by an outgoing, petite woman with wavy, shoulder-length russet hair and a luminous smile. She looked like someone I might sit next to at an art museum lecture. "I'm Cheryl Grigorian," she said. "They call me Dr. G."

She showed me into an examining room. An x-ray machine hovered above a table. Dr. G. said the machine would show her where to insert a needle through which she would withdraw tissue. She would numb me with morphine; I would not feel pain. Despite her reassurance, a long needle jammed into my hipbone sounded like a POW torture technique. I asked for a sedative. She gave me a Versed I.V.

As Dr. G. pushed, I closed my eyes. To my relief, she was right. I felt pressure but no pain. I told her about my book, and we chatted like girlfriends. Dr. G. agreed to let us wait while she delivered the tissue sample to a nearby pathologist. I sat jiggling my foot. Several minutes later, Dr. G. returned. When I saw her face, my spirits collapsed. There were tears in her eyes.

"The lesion appears to be metastatic adenocarcinoma," she said.

"Malignant?" I whispered.

She nodded.

Life had turned into a series of waiting. Waiting in lobbies and examining rooms. Waiting to take tests. Waiting to hear results. Two days later, I underwent a brain MRI (magnetic resonance image) which visualizes the brain without using x-ray. I lay on a padded table which pulled me into a narrow tunnel, the center of a large circular magnet. The headphones gripping my ears did little to muffle loud banging noises. Burton sat at the end of the table, holding my foot, making both of us feel a little less vulnerable.

Later, I sat outside the nuclear medicine department waiting for a PET (positron emission tomography) scan. *Here we are again,* I wrote in my journal, *waiting. This time for a scan I hear costs $5,000. Thank God for Blue Cross.*

A nurse led me into another examining room. Matt, thin with a grey ponytail, gave me an intravenous injection of Tc-99m, or Technium 99, a radioactive isotope with a sugar base. It accumulates in the presence of malignancies and shows up as hot spots. A PET scan can detect malignancies the size of a pin head.

I lay on a table on my back, then stomach, as Matt operated a gamma camera that moved along my body, three inches a minute. It took three hours to photograph me from the base of my skull to my upper thighs. I prayed and drifted in and out.

David accompanied us that day. I was grateful to have him along. He could make me smile in the bleakest times, and Burton needed support as well.

After my PET scan, David asked, "What did they find, Mom?"

"I don't know," I said.

"You and dad get the car. I'll catch up with you."

We had been at the hospital so long that the front door had closed. Our car had been moved to another lot. As we trudged down a long hallway toward the other exit, we heard David's voice from behind.

"Mom, Dad, wait," he called. We turned to see him sprinting toward us, muscular from the tennis he played. Fortunately both of our sons had their father's athletic ability. A grin beamed from David's suntanned face as though he had just aced a serve.

"Good news, Mom," he said, fidgeting with a string—a habit of his since he was a little boy. "Other than the pelvis, your bones are clear."

"How do you know?"

"I tracked down Matt and bugged him into telling me. I'm so relieved, Mom. I had begun to feel like we were the Bad News Bears. I expected Walter Matthau to walk around the corner."

"Walter Matthau is dead," Burton said.

David said, "No wonder he didn't show up."

I felt an odd sensation bubble up within me. It was the first time I laughed in days.

No matter how many friends and relatives you have lost to cancer or how many terrifying statistics you have read, your brain resists a cancer diagnosis. Dr. G. had said, "appears to be." She hadn't said, "is." I thought I knew my body. My body wouldn't do this to me. *Despite the evidence,* I wrote, *part of me still believes this is all a big overreaction.*

Two weeks had passed since the MRI that showed probable cancer in my pelvis. We still did not know where the trouble, whatever it was, had started. Dr. Jack Ruckdeschel, Karmanos president and chief executive officer, agreed to help us make sense of my case.

Dr. R. was a big, genial bear of a man. His blue eyes looked even bluer against the sky outside the windows of his spacious corner office. He leaned forward in his white lab coat and patted a large hand on the desk. "Let me tell you something about cancer."

A tumor begins with one dysplastic or pre-malignant cell, he said. He drew circles on a legal pad, starting with a dot, followed by progressively larger circles. By the time a lesion shows on a scan, one cell has multiplied into over one billion cells and is slightly smaller than a dime. A lesion doubles in size in three to six months.

My eyes strayed to the aquamarine sky; my mind followed, wishing I were on the golf course, even four-putting. Dr. R. continued. I willed my hand to race along the pages of my journal.

Two masses in my pelvis surrounded and pressed on my uterus and bladder, he said. Two expanding black holes had taken over my pelvic bones. A lesion in my throat, one to one and a half centimeters, covered most of the right side of my thyroid. They had ruled out cancer of the lung, breast, pancreas, kidney, liver, colon and rectum, he said. I silently thanked each organ he named.

How tied we are to our bodies, I thought. When they work, we are blissfully unaware of them. Now, a large stranger in a white coat knew more about my insides than I did. I wished I could separate myself from my body, withdraw my soul or essence or whatever it was that made me, me, and keep it somewhere safe, in some celestial vault, while doctors put the rest back in order, returned me to health, so I could go on hugging my husband, smelling my granddaughter's hair, improving my putting stroke—ordinary things that had never seemed so extraordinary.

"The pathologist thinks you have adenocarcinoma," Dr. R. said. "He's running the stains to make sure. We will come up with a proper diagnosis—cancer of the thyroid, ovaries, uterus or bladder. Or a carcinoma of an unknown primary. Each type has a different treatment."

Dr. R. had scheduled me for an ultra-sound guided needle biopsy of my thyroid that afternoon. "That will help us know if we are looking at one cancer or two. Whatever, we'll deal with it. Right now I'm more concerned about the masses in your pelvis pressing on your bladder. They could block your ureter and restrict your ability to urinate."

Great, I thought. Something else to worry about.

Drumming my fingers on the table, I said, "I'm feeling really anxious. The only way I've been getting through this is with Xanax."

"Xanax is Vitamin X," he said. "It takes the edge off." He scribbled on a prescription pad, tore off the page and handed it to me.

"Here's a script for a stronger dose. Take whatever you need. I'd also like you to put on some weight before surgery and chemo. What you need now is calories and joy. Whatever joy means to you. To me, it's an apple martini and a steak.

"In fighting cancer, your first chance is your best chance. If we think your cancer is curable, we'll recommend more toxicity up front. If not, we'll take a more moderate approach."

I caught my breath. "Curable?" I repeated. Hope nudged the boulder lodged in my belly. "Is that possible?"

He nodded and smiled. "We cure lots of cancers today."

CHAPTER 4

Counting on Miracles

It's these turnaround or pivotal moments that introduce you to yourself...these small or huge catastrophic events in your life—I do think that's where you really meet yourself.

—Sheryl Crow, *O, The Oprah Magazine*

I HAD BEEN away from our farmhouse for twelve days. My powder blue crew neck sweater lay in the sink where I left it. I had planned to wash it in Woolite two days later when I returned, after receiving an MRI of my pelvis and a prescription for osteoporosis pills. When I left the farmhouse that Sunday morning in late July, I was a different person. A healthy person with a pulled groin and a balsamic vinaigrette-stained sweater.

Now I felt weak, fearful and no longer able to trust my body. I had always been irrational about the prospect of cancer. I didn't wear t-shirts adorned with pink ribbons, lest "the girls" be reminded. Ditto, lapel pins. I gave away golf balls printed with pink ribbons. I grew up calling cancer the C-word. The thought that the C-word might, though I still didn't believe it, have infested part of me twisted my stomach. I prayed over and over that it wasn't so.

Being back up north meant a brief break from doctors' appointments and medical tests and the malaise of dread. Sore as I was, I needed exercise. Burton did, too. I was desperate to do something normal.

On Saturday morning, I asked, "How about a bike ride?"

A smile spread across Burton's face.

Burton loaded our bikes into the bed of our black Chevy Silverado. We drove to downtown Charlevoix and picked up sandwiches at Scovie's. We took off on the bike trail along Lake Michigan toward Petoskey. Forward motion didn't hurt. I was glad to peddle without pain. I focused on the sun warming my shoulders, the breeze cooling my face, the fragrance of evergreens and, in the off chance the suspicion of cancer proved right, Dr. R's promise that some tumors were curable.

Reaching a small public beach, we sat at a picnic table admiring clear, turquoise water. For several summers when our sons were young we joined friends here, on what used to be called Elzinga Beach, for a cookout. We roasted hotdogs and marshmallows on sticks. As the sun settled into the lake, we bit into juicy slabs of watermelon and held contests spitting the brown seeds. These were the days before seedless watermelons, which are more eater-friendly but useless for producing spit-worthy missiles. David and Andy argued over whose seed sailed farthest.

"The boys always ended up spitting seeds at each other and pushing each other around," I said. "I worried so much about their fighting."

"Today they're best friends," Burton said.

Burton bent down to pick some wild daisies and grasses. He wedged them through a crack in the table. "Now it's a party."

I ate chicken salad on multigrain bread; Burton, an Italian sub with salami and cheese. I had given up encouraging Burton to eat healthier. He knew what was and wasn't good for him, and I didn't want to nag.

We talked about how Lake Michigan had receded. Thirty years ago, few rocks peeked from the water. Now hundreds popped up along the shoreline. I suggested global warming was responsible. Burton said the lake rose and fell in natural cycles and that nature fights back. Disease commandeers your head as well as your body. I was conscious of the effort it took to hold a normal conversation.

Burton helped me over some boulders. When we reached one large enough for both of us, Burton sat beside me, rubbing my shoulders. My tense muscles loosened under his strong hands. I listened to waves lap against the shore, watched them rise and melt. A few years back, at the height of our problems, Burton disappeared for many hours at a stretch. Lately, he had scarcely left my side. My precarious condition had made both of us aware of what we could lose.

"I hate to admit this," I said. "The old me wouldn't have appreciated this as much."

"Let's pray," Burton said. We bowed our heads.

For most of my life, I didn't believe in God. God didn't make sense, and as a girl, I rejected what didn't make sense. I was raised as a Reform Jew. That meant ducking out of Sunday school services when I could and anointing myself, instead, with Almond Joys and Good & Plentys in the nearby candy store. It meant attending services as a family on Yom Kippur and, in December, a menorah in the kitchen and a Christmas tree in the living room. I wasn't adamant enough to call myself an atheist, but I deemed needing God for weaklings. I wanted to depend on myself.

When I was fifteen, my father, then in his late thirties, decided to convert. He was suffering business reversals at the time. When Dad returned from World War II, he had gone into the blueprint business with his father. (The business had been started by his mother, Mollie, whose brother was architect Albert Kahn. Mollie retired to raise children. She died when I was a baby.) In 1956, Dad's father and stepmother, flying home from vacationing in California, were killed in a United Airlines midair plane collision above the Grand Canyon. Dad took over the company. Competition was fierce, upgrading equipment was expensive, and Dad struggled. He longed for spiritual support he didn't find in Judaism. He told my mother, sister and me he had decided to seek another religion. No big deal, I thought. He'll become Unitarian. I knew and liked several Unitarians at my school. But Dad had bigger plans. On a business trip, he picked up a Gideon's bible and experienced a vision of Jesus. He returned home and became Catholic. He disappeared to church every Sunday morning, joined a prayer group and left cross-emblazoned pamphlets on the seat of his car that, as I used to say, gave me the creeps. People are far more accepting of changing religions today. At the time, Dad's conversion was a scandal, the talk of our Jewish circle. Mom tried to be understanding, but I could tell she was embarrassed. I was, too. I saw my father's conversion as a sign of weakness. It would be many years before I understood the courage it must have taken.

Soon after Dad became Catholic, our family went skiing up north at Boyne Mountain. On a chairlift, I met a boy from Saginaw. He had short straw colored hair, white teeth and a firm jaw and was so cute that I found myself nodding when he invited me to accompany him to Christmas mass. On the way out of the service, among the crowd of rosary-carrying, veil-wearing worshippers, I spotted my father. I can still feel the heat of my cringe as I ducked my head and veered the other way.

Agnosticism accompanied me into my fifties, a time when I became depressed by my mother's health problems. Mom was wheelchair-bound, reclusive and dependent on aides. I would run ads and call agencies and interview and hire aides for her; within days, she would fire them. I became so discouraged by my inability to improve life for my mother that I began drinking too much. When friends asked about her, I'd say, "I'm not getting drinker's elbow for nothing." Burton grew impatient with my complaining. One night, in desperation, I prayed for what may have been twenty or thirty minutes for release from my worries. I awoke the next morning with a new sensation. I felt physically lighter.

Not long after God helped me with my mother problem, I needed God again. The marriage I had counted on began to crumble. Prayer made me feel a little less alone. It gave me the courage to seek counseling. Burton and I attended a couples' program, admitted the trouble we were in and began praying together. Prayer pulled us through some painful times. It helped us to forgive—each other and ourselves. It showed us that something bigger was in charge. Slowly, hard work, underscored by prayer, mended the tear in our relationship, darned us back together like a pair of old socks. Fears for my marriage gradually dissolved.

Now, I had strayed into an even scarier place. I needed God more than ever. Fear of losing my husband was replaced by an even bigger fear. As much as prayer consoled me, my fears ran deeper still. It would be a while before I could begin to let them go, before I sensed the many ways God would show up in my life.

At twenty, our friend and rabbi Daniel Syme was diagnosed with a rare form of potentially fatal testicular cancer. Now, over forty years later, Danny visited us at home in Franklin. I asked him to tell me the story of his illness.

He told me how he wasn't expected to survive; how his cancer type was so virulent that if a single cell had escaped the tumor, he would have died. He told me that ten years later he learned that only one person with the same disease was known to have survived as long as six months.

He underwent two surgeries. The first, to remove and biopsy the tumor. A second exploratory surgery took five hours with two surgeons. After that operation, one of his surgeons reported back to him. Danny's tumor had been totally encapsulated. The surgeon, also Jewish, told him he had expected to find that the tumor had spread. "But I didn't find anything," he said. He added, "In my opinion, you should become a rabbi. There's something you're supposed to do."

Danny, whose father was a rabbi, said, "At the time, I was planning to go into psychology or law. I listened to my doctor and switched to rabbinical school. I try to live each day doing something of value, in the hope that somehow, at some point, I've done the thing I was supposed to do."

Visiting me, I was sure, was among the things he was supposed to do. I felt better just hearing his story. I felt better when he promised to repeat my name during religious services when the *mishe-beirach*, or Jewish healing prayer, was read.

"It's best to speak your Hebrew name," he said.

"I don't think I have one."

"I thought you might not. I decided on one for you: Ariella Chava, Lioness of God."

"Lioness," I repeated and blinked back tears. "I feel more like a helpless cub."

"I did, too."

Wearing a dark grey suit instead of the white robe he wore on the *bimah*, Danny still exuded a gentle authority. He placed his hands on my head, spoke my new name and said a prayer for me in Hebrew. As he turned to walk out the door, he stopped and gazed at me.

"Ariella Chava," he said. "You're going to be fine. In my line of work, I don't just hope for miracles. I count on them."

Ellen was one of dozens of people who called to check on me. Having faced down breast cancer, Ellen asked, "What stage are you? The stage where it kinda sucks? It sorta sucks? Or it totally sucks?" Ellen sent me a little book that had helped her, *There's No Place Like Hope*. She tabbed several pages and starred her favorite passages.

I was amazed at how attentive people were, especially since when my controversial first book came out, all but my closest friends scurried away. Cards and gifts and calls flooded in. Lisa sent a different Beanie Baby bear every week. A bigger bear, dark brown and a foot tall, came from Andy's friend Jon. Chemo Bear had accompanied Jon through months of grueling but successful treatment for advanced testicular cancer.

Marilyn brought a soft, tan, stuffed teddy bear wearing a t-shirt with the *mishe-beirach* printed on the back. Mishe Bear became my constant bedtime companion. Burton deemed him his competition. As a youngster, I'd had a stuffed black-and-white dog I called Doggie. Not giving him a real name made it seem less babyish to sleep with him every night. Doggie became more and more threadbare until I had to sew his ear back on. In my mid-teens, my mother convinced me to store him in an old, brown-and-white plaid Saks box in the basement, along with the foreign dolls my grandmother had brought back from her travels. Four-and-a-half decades later, I justified sleeping with Mishe Bear because he wore the Jewish healing prayer on his t-shirt and I wanted God to remember how desperately I longed to be well.

Another Marilyn gave me a Native American Wisdom Stone, meant to be placed under my pillow at night to encourage dreams and keep me in touch with my inner wisdom. Susu, a breast cancer survivor, brought me a silver bracelet interlaced with red string, a symbol of *Kabbalah*, the tradition of Jewish mysticism. "For luck," she said as she fastened it around my wrist. Sandy researched alternative therapies on the Internet and sent us Web sites. She delivered homemade lentil soup and an encyclopedia on medicine. Sally brought over red boxing gloves symbolizing my need to fight.

Brenda laminated a card. The front, labeled Ariella, showed a photo of a lioness. She had taken the picture on a trip to Africa. On the back, she printed the *mishe-beirach*. Jeanie brought me back a Lord Ganesha from India. "He's the remover of obstacles," she said. The card and the icon still reside on a shelf by my bed. Mishe Bear still presides over my pillow.

At any given moment I either felt strengthened by so much support or terrified that people must really think I was a goner.

Part of me still refused to concede I had cancer. Despite the evidence, I grasped at other theories the way fasting Jews pounce on Yom Kippur supper.

Dr. Ira Mickelson (Dr. Mike), my regular gynecologist, had performed a pelvic exam on me six months before, and found nothing wrong. Now he speculated I might have benign bilateral fibroid tumors along with bone lesions I'd had for years. Most ovarian tumors were benign, Dr. Mike promised.

My brother-in-law Neal, a retired orthopedist, proposed a diagnosis called osteitis fibrosa cystica, or Von Recklinghausen's disease. It was a form of hyperparathryroidism. It sounded grim. But not as grim as cancer.

Burton and I needed a night off. As long as I babied my left leg, I felt fine. If I were on a fast track to meet my maker, I didn't want to look back and know I'd wasted a glorious summer night worrying about matters we couldn't control.

"Let's go on a date," I said.

Burton's face brightened. "Great idea."

Business took Andy all over the city, so I asked him to recommend a restaurant. "Somewhere romantic," I said. I think special occasions are more memorable when celebrated someplace new. This wasn't a birthday or anniversary, but it was an occasion.

Burton put down the top of our black Thunderbird. We drove only black cars, a less-than-intelligent preference as we lived on dirt roads downstate and up north. But Burton washed the car in the driveway in honor of our date, and off we went. I determined to believe in Neal's osteitis diagnosis and to enjoy my husband's company. I didn't give a thought to my flailing hair as we drove some fifteen miles across town to Andy's recommendation—a place with no memories of happier times, where we were unlikely to run into anyone who might ask about my health.

Fonte d'Amore turned out to be a cozy spot with white tablecloths, low lighting and a few other diners, none familiar. In one corner, a black singer with the surprising name of James

Cohen accompanied himself on a piano. He had a fine, deep voice and sang "Rambling Rose" and "It's All in the Game." We drank red wine and savored sublime calamari fried with semi-hot peppers. My taste buds did not realize they were hovering on the brink of death.

Burton clinked my glass with our usual toast. "Good health. Long life."

"To Von Recklinghausen," I said.

I had resolved not to cry, and I didn't—all the way to the cappuccino and the first notes of "Send in the Clowns," a song that undoes me every time.

On our way out, we stopped to tell the entertainer how much we'd enjoyed his music. Burton put ten dollars into the glass bowl on the piano and also bought a CD. I resisted the urge to tell my husband that five dollars would have been a perfectly nice tip. I knew what he'd say from the many times I hadn't mustered such restraint. He'd say, "Five dollars means more to him than it does to me." And he'd add, "If ten dollars is going to break me, I might as well be broke." James Cohen and the night breeze serenaded us all the way home.

That night and the next day I clung to my hope that my brother-in-law's theory would prove correct. Two days later, my sister-in-law dropped by.

"By the way," Anita said. At times, Anita has the subtlety of an earthquake. "David drove over to our house with your x-rays. Neal looked at them and decided there was no chance his osteitis theory could apply."

David, who knew I was rooting for osteitis, hadn't mentioned the visit.

At thirty-six, Ginger was diagnosed with MS. We had talked about her illness a few years before, briefly. I kept all such conversations brief. Worrier that I was, I figured the less I knew about a problem, the less chance I'd develop it. Now I wanted to know how my friend, almost twenty years younger than I, had coped so gracefully.

"It is what it is," she said on the phone. "Sometimes my hand works and sometimes it decides to spill hot coffee. I clean up and move on. I took about a year to come to terms with my illness. I had to grieve the loss of who I was and accept who I needed to become. I learned to be more protective of my time and my body, to save my energy for what mattered, and not to push myself. I learned to rest. When you first hear bad news, you have no idea how you'll get through it. But you do. You build in things to look forward to."

To help her heal, Ginger and husband Ken built a labyrinth behind their home in northern Michigan. "It symbolizes life's journeys, inside and out," Ginger said. "We made the aisles wide enough for a wheelchair, in case I ever need one." I marveled at the calm in her voice.

My friend Gertrude once ran a contemporary art gallery in Detroit. In her nineties, she had had two open-heart surgeries and a hip replacement. When I asked how she remained so young in spirit, she said, "I focus on the things I can do; not on the things I can't." Ginger lived the same philosophy.

Ginger invited me to walk her labyrinth. "It will help you learn to trust the universe."

Days later, back up north, I drove to Petoskey. Ginger directed me to her labyrinth. She told me to expect a surprise in the middle and to help myself when I found it. I followed the edge of a flower bed up a gradual slope and turned into a clearing. My skin prickled to see curved ridges covered with cosmos, daisies, black-eyed Susans and grasses. In the distance, Lake Michigan glistened in the sunlight.

I strolled through the aisles, following openings that led to the center. With each step, I touched my thumb to the tip of a finger, from index to pinkie, one at a time. It was a ritual I once learned from a healer friend Rita, walking a different labyrinth. I repeated "*sa ta na ma*," Sanskrit for "I dwell in God's truth." I also prayed for a return to health and for the strength to weather the days ahead.

Atop a small stand in the center was a clear glass bowl labeled Pearls of Wisdom. The bowl was filled with iridescent glass bubbles. Scattered among them were several tiny tubes of paper tied with pale blue, satin ribbons. I picked out one little scroll, opened it and caught my breath. At the time, I didn't realize that little miracles like this would keep happening. I only knew this scrap of paper comforted me.

> Ask, and it shall be given you; seek, and ye shall find; knock, and it shall be opened unto you. (Matthew 7:7)

I floated back to Ginger's house, found my friend and unfolded my fingers around the message cradled in my hand.

"Were there lots of messages in that bowl?" I asked.

"Lots," she said. For a party the night before, she had filled the bowl with dozens of her favorite quotes. Most had already been picked.

"Yours just happened to be left."

I lay beside Burton, trying not to shift my weight. Whenever I turned, pain stabbed me in the groin, reminding me, as if I needed reminding, of how careless I'd been, how I wished I had taken the pain seriously right away. I had taped my biblical message into my journal and tried to hang on to the sense of calm I received from Ginger's labyrinth, but the feeling ebbed. Fear oozed back into the spaces between my vertebrae.

We had seen or spoken to several doctors. No one could give us a definite diagnosis. That day we had visited another gynecological oncologist, this one at Beaumont Hospital. Another set of stirrups, another cold metal speculum, another latex glove probing inside me. After, in his office, Dr. Sheldon Weiner had told me my masses appeared to be mobile, not stuck to the bone. He said this in a positive tone, as if it were good news.

Against all odds, I still hoped I didn't have cancer. I crossed my fingers. "Could the masses be benign?" I asked.

"They could," he said. My fingers tightened. "I doubt it." My hand went limp.

For years, I had kept journals. I recorded details of vacations, of Burton's business deals. I wrote about my worries. I wrote about things my children said or did. About the time David, age eight, peed into the favorite drinking cup of his best friend, Josh's, sister Karen. (Burton dismissed it as a meaningless prank; I feared it signaled a lack of concern for others.) About my panic when Andy, leading a high school group of younger students on a spring camping trip in the Smoky Mountains, got stuck in what was called the Storm of the Century. ("Don't worry," Burton said. "He's trained for this." Andy had completed a program with the National Outdoor Leadership School. Still, I carried on to such an extent that Burton called information and got the numbers of every ranger's station in the park and phoned them all, finally reaching a ranger at the last number. He assured us everyone would be fine. After a few hours, Andy led his group through waist-deep snow and out of the park to safety.)

Given my lack of control over what was happening in my life, taking notes helped me feel I was doing something productive. I filled my journal with doctors' phone numbers and comments and tabbed the pages—orange for numbers, yellow for comments. I wrote out scriptures and affirmations and marked those pages with pink tabs. I jotted down any hopeful medical mention. There weren't enough of those to merit a colored tab. We would not begin to hear any truly hopeful news until three weeks after my internist first voiced concern. When the diagnosis might be cancer, three weeks is eternity.

I laid my journal on the bed and looked at my husband. He jabbed at the remote control, staring at the TV. Sections of the *Detroit News* were strewn around him. A pair of wire glasses lay on the legal pad beside him. Burton regularly misplaced his reading glasses and bought new ones with wire or plastic frames by the dozen at the Dollar Store. I thought about how hard Burton had been working. A friend who had helped his wife through breast cancer advised him, "Be diligent." He had initiated endless calls and, despite his ADD, had done his best not to lose the notes. That day he had spoken to five doctors.

I patted the legal pad. "Thank you," I murmured.

Burton turned to me. "Don't thank me. I'm doing this for us. You're not just a part of my life. You *are* my life. For the last three weeks, I lost the desire to eat or talk to friends or read the paper. I'd be in a public place and look around and think: How could people not know my wife could die soon, my world has stopped? I've prayed for the best but worried about the worst. These three weeks have been torture. I've been in free fall."

He put up his hand. "It's time to stop," he said.

"I believe we'll get through this. Imagine we own a real estate deal that's pumping out cash. The tenant is AAA. Right this minute, you and I are that kind of deal. I've been letting myself get depressed, wondering what I'd do without you. I've taken Xanax to get through the days and Ambien to sleep at night. It's time for a new attitude. You're here. We're together now. That's what matters. Let's enjoy every minute."

He stretched out his right arm. I leaned my head against his neck. He smelled of cinnamon.

"I didn't always realize it, but now I know I'm the luckiest guy in the world to have you. I love coming home to you. I love having you come home to me. I love walking with you and paddling with you in a canoe. I love your wisdom. I'm sorry for any time I took you for granted."

We had lived a miracle. The struggle to save our marriage had deepened our appreciation for each other. We had worked so hard to overcome one crisis only to be met with another. It didn't seem fair. I was sucking on self-pity like menthol cough drops. Several years before, Andy, a high school senior, was playing football. Cranbrook was competing against arch-rival Country Day. Late in the game, Andy's teammate and best friend, Roger, a running back, was carrying the ball, bound for the end zone. A touch down would have given Cranbrook the lead and their first potential victory against Country Day in many years. An out-of-bounds flag was thrown. Burton and I were sitting at the point of the supposed foul and were certain Roger's feet remained inside the line. Cranbrook lost another game to Country Day. After, I was fuming about the injustice. Andy said, "Let it go, Mom. Life isn't always fair."

Now I faced a new challenge—to cut the self-pity. To trust my healing to God and modern medicine. And to my husband who, despite our recent travails, was determined to make me well. I lay with my head on Burton's chest. His pajama top grew moist.

"I'm sorry, too," I said, "for any time I was distracted or too busy to listen. For any time I didn't stop to appreciate you. Let's pray for more than ninety days."

I kept trying to talk myself out of having cancer. The delusion was getting harder to pull off. I felt grateful to have a retreat 200-plus miles away from hospitals and doctors and dire prognoses.

In early August, we again escaped north for the weekend. At our farmhouse, I went through the motions of a normal, healthy person. I sliced and sautéed Vidalia onions and Portobello mushrooms, took out a pan, poured in olive oil, turned on a gas burner. Burton grilled rib eye steaks—amazingly tender, from Sam's Club—marinated in soy sauce and olive oil.

Burton pulled out an expensive Caymus Reserve. I raised my eyebrows.

"What are we waiting for?" he said.

Jim and Nancy joined us for dinner. Jim was a psychologist who had written a blurb for my book. Nancy, an artist. They were empathetic, positive people—the only kind of people I could bear being with in my frayed emotional state.

Later, our friend Eric stopped by. In summer, Eric held campfire sing-a-longs for our family and friends. He wrote a ballad for Burton's sixtieth birthday a year before and had since written one for mine. With chilly weather earlier in the summer and my illness later, Eric hadn't had a chance to sing my song for me. I asked to hear it.

He pulled his guitar strap over his head. "I feel kind of funny singing this now," he said. "It's called 'Suzy Lights up the Town.'" As I listened to Eric's mellow, smoky voice sing about me in better times, I bit my lip. I wondered if I'd ever light up any place again.

Eric sang a few more songs we loved, including "My Heroes Have Always Been Cowboys" and "Country Road." I asked him to sing "Amazing Grace." He had never sung a hymn for us before, but he was a part-time minister so I figured he'd know it. His delivery resonated through me.

Eric slowed his tempo for the final "but now I see." He slipped the worn strap over his head. As he started to put his guitar back in the case, he paused. "I'll do one more," he said and put the strap back on.

Remembering the message I'd received on my walk through Ginger's labyrinth, I felt goose bumps rise on my arms. Eric sang a hymn I had never heard before: "Ask and Ye Shall Receive."

We were scheduled to fly to New York for a second opinion at Memorial Sloan-Kettering Hospital. I wondered how anyone could come up with a helpful second opinion when we still lacked a clear first opinion.

Still up north, Burton and I visited the lake about half a mile from our farmhouse. We watched sunlight dance on the water, a sight so pretty my heart ached. We drove back home to check for messages. None.

As we were about to leave, an unfamiliar car pulled into the driveway. Dr. Mike and his wife, Linda, got out. Dr. Mike was my gynecologist of several years. He was short and smiley, a panda bear. I had visited him for my annual check-up six months before. Nothing appeared wrong. Recently, he had been helping us interpret medical findings.

Dr. Mike and Linda happened to be visiting Michigania, a camp for U OF M alumni, about an hour's drive away. "We tried to call, but our cell phone didn't get through," Dr. Mike said. "We took a chance and came anyway."

"I'm so glad you did," I said, hugging him. "Two minutes later, we'd have been gone again."

We sat on the porch sipping lemonade. Dr. Mike reached into his pocket, pulled out a heart-shaped Petoskey stone, and handed it to me. "For luck," he said. "I carved and polished it myself at camp." Petoskey stones are unique to northern Michigan. Fossilized coral about 350 million years old, they bear small round marks resembling cells. I have loved rocks since I was a girl. I no longer possessed my childhood collection of mineral specimens. But now I had a more meaningful one.

Cancer messes with your head as well as your body. As I stroked the cool, mottled stone, I had a *Course in Miracles* moment. There were two ways to see Dr. Mike's gift. Fear-based: He's worried I might sue him for not detecting my cancer in January. Loving: He cares about me and feels terrible that my cancer wasn't detectable in January. The *Course* says we choose how we see things.

"It's beautiful," I said.

"What's the latest?"

"We've seen a lot of doctors. We still don't know my primary. It might be uterine."

"Uterine cancer generally occurs in overweight women," he said. Fat cells produce estrogen, which thickens the walls of the uterus. Early on, the condition is pre-cancerous and well-differentiated. Adenocarcinoma occurs over time. It can be detected by scraping cells from the lining of the uterus in a procedure called a dilation and curettage.

"Have you had a D&C?"

"No."

Dr. Malone had wanted to perform a hysterectomy right away, I explained, which would have negated the need for a D&C. When we held off on the hysterectomy to consult with bone and other specialists, we missed what I now realized was a logical step. Coming up with a cancer diagnosis is seldom clear cut. The discovery period can be long and confusing. As diligent as we had tried to be, we had not been diligent enough.

"Come to my office Monday at seven. You'll be my first patient."

Two mornings later I lay on Dr. Mike's table. I was grateful for his prompt attention if not for the cramping in my uterus. "Almost done," Dr. Mike said. From between my legs, he muttered, "I'm getting a lot of gritty tissue. I think this is your primary."

Burton and I drove to Karmanos to drop off my uterine tissue sample. It was a surreal feeling knowing we carried evidence that could reveal my fate, and that it sat in a small, harmless-looking cardboard box on my lap.

We stopped at a traffic light. I noticed an NAI/Farbman for-sale sign in front of a nearby office building. Our white, red and black real-estate signs bloomed around the city. A fog of fear and lethargy had surrounded me since the day I first heard the word "lesions." I made a conscious effort to pay attention to something other than my troubles.

"I still enjoy seeing our signs," I said. I refrained from droning on about how many more I might get to see.

"Until they're marked SOLD, they just represent overhead," Burton said.

"You worked really hard to bring the company to the point where the boys would want to take over."

"You've always been my best cheerleader," Burton said. "You enrich my life. I need at least twenty-five more years of enrichment."

"Sign me up."

"We've been together most of our lives. That's worth fighting for. I'm up for the fight. We'll get all the reinforcements we need and move forward. We've got the best medical team in the country, so much love from family and friends, and God is our quarterback. How do you beat that?"

Again I felt grateful I hadn't given up on our marriage. And grateful Burton hadn't given up on me. I unbuckled my seatbelt and leaned over and kissed my husband's rosy, upper cheek. "You don't."

Back home, we called Karmanos. The tissue from my D&C had been analyzed. I did, in fact, have cancer in the epithelial lining of my uterus. Uterine cancer, as Dr. Mike predicted. Dr. Mike's unexpected appearance at the farm two days before was another coincidence I would come to see as more than a coincidence. At the time, I just considered it a lucky break.

The cancer experience is full of ups and downs. I appreciated the medical attention I was receiving. I was relieved to know the primary source, or mostly relieved. Until that moment, a stubborn shoot in my heart refused to surrender. A tiny part of me still hoped the experts were wrong, that I didn't have the dreaded C-word.

There was no more room for denial.

CHAPTER 5

Nowhere to Hide

I'm a writer, for better or worse, and when the universe hands you material like this, not writing about it seems either a waste or a conscious act of evasion.

—Christopher Buckley, *Losing Mum and Pup*

PEOPLE KEPT TURNING up to help me navigate the strange, frightening world into which I had strayed. Jill was a psychologist and friend. She was also the wife of our rabbi and friend, Danny. Though they took different approaches, they were both committed to providing spiritual support. Their dual disciplines complemented each other and showed what I was beginning to learn, that wisdom comes from diverse traditions. And that I could take advantage of all of them. Jill tried to help me glimpse past the fear that walled in my days and nights. One afternoon shortly before my surgery, she joined me on our back porch.

There's something special about a porch. It connects us with nature yet shelters us, too. Ours has a cathedral ceiling, exposed rafters, screens on three sides and juts into treetops. It has verdigris wrought-iron chairs, a table and a loveseat decorated with seahorses, all of which belonged to my grandmother. (I began calling her *grand-mère* when I started studying French in middle school. Paris was her favorite city.) *Grand-mère* and

I used to sit on the loveseat and nibble cheese wafers, watching small cars below on the John Lodge expressway. High on the terrace of her apartment at North Park Towers in nearby Southfield, I felt safe and adored. *Grand-mère*, who died when I was in my late twenties, wore suits from Oscar de la Renta and Pauline Trigère. (Irresistible aside: In the three decades I wrote about fashion, my favorite fashion-related story concerned American designer Pauline Trigère. She was lunching with my once-publisher John Fairchild at La Grenouille in New York. A diner approached them and told Ms. Trigère how his mother had loved her clothes, and how she was buried wearing one of her suits. When the diner left the table, Ms. Trigère turned to Fairchild and said, "As I was saying, in a Trigère, you can go anywhere.") My grandmother was, to me, the essence of refinement and good taste. (She was buried in an Oscar.)

Although dust from the dirt road drifted in, the porch remained my favorite part of the house. But today my knees jiggled. I felt neither safe nor sheltered.

"People keep telling me to be positive," I said. "I want to think good thoughts. I try to think good thoughts. But I'm so afraid."

Jill had dark brown hair cropped short like a boy's and the cheekbones to carry it off. She was as direct and no-nonsense as her hairstyle. She looked at me with penetrating hazel eyes.

"Everything in life is faith or fear," she said. "Your life is not in the hands of this illness. It's in the hands of the Divine. The universe gives us the lessons we need. To get you through your habit of negative thinking, the universe has given you its toughest lesson."

Jill knew I was a chronic worrier. Sitting beside me on a swing that hangs from a rafter, she pulled a deck of colorful cards from her bag. She fanned them out on the glass-topped table in front of us. Each pictured a different character.

"Each card shows an archetype, a part of our personality," Jill said. "Pick the ones that speak to you."

I pointed to several, including the Warrior, the Hero, the Hermit and the Chronicler. Jill put away the others and spread the cards I had chosen on the table.

"The Warrior means you're a fighter," Jill said. "You stand up for your beliefs. You fight for your health. The Hero shows your desire to help others. The Hermit represents your need for time to yourself—something all women need. The Chronicler is the part of you who writes about your struggles."

My knees continued to shake. "What about my Chicken?" I asked. "How do I get through the fear?"

"Two little vowels are all that come between worrier and warrior," Jill said. "It's natural to feel fear. You feel it and keep going. Your challenge now is to befriend yourself."

I loathed the turbulence fear caused in my gut and tried to avoid fearful situations. On some occasions I forced myself to push past my fears.

We're all influenced by the times in which we are raised. The 1950s were an era of conformity. Most women stayed home and raised children. Betty Friedan's *The Feminine Mystique,* published in 1963, cast light on the dissatisfaction many women felt with the role of full-time housewife, something I never wanted to be. I admired Betty Friedan. And Gloria Steinem, another fighter. As a young journalist, Steinem impersonated a Playboy Bunny and wrote a searing magazine article about women as sex objects. She campaigned for the Equal Rights Amendment. While a reporter for the *Detroit News,* I interviewed Gloria. As reticent as I found her, I was awed by the courage of this Jewish girl from Toledo, Ohio (just a few miles from Detroit), 10 years older than I was.

The Roman god Janus has two faces, looking in opposite directions. I had two faces, too—one on the surface, the other, within. The outside conformist wanted acceptance; the inside rebel, to express herself. One sunny spring day in college at the University of Michigan, I gave vent to my inside rebel. I attended Music Lit class wearing a yellow, rubber rain slicker with nothing underneath. For me, it represented a private act of defiance. Small as it was, I felt brave and a little giddy. And proud of my courage.

There were other times when I pushed conventional limits and forced myself past my fears. In the first gossip column I wrote for the *Detroit News*, I revealed the secret of John Delorean's facelift. Delorean was then a glamorous, admired top executive of General Motors. The item launched my column as a must-read phenomenon. Writing about our marriage problems was another act of boldness—some would say insanity. But it was therapy for me and for many readers.

Beneath such acts of daring, I still felt like a frightened little girl trying to be brave. I was still the eleven-year-old troubled by the silences and arguments between her parents. The eleven-year-old who sat in her room, with her doll collection in the corner cupboard and the raggedy, stuffed dog on her bed, who ignored the churning in her belly and said to her mother, "If you're not happy with Dad, leave him."

Nearly fifty years later, I was still that anxious little girl, tamping down fear with attempted courage. The effort was exhausting. And now I felt fear of a different kind. Fear not due to anything I wrote or did or said, but to something bigger, beyond my control. Something that had blindsided me.

Burton joined us on the porch and sat in one of my grandmother's chairs.

"How are you doing?" Jill asked.

"I believe Suzy's going to make it." Burton pumped his fist. "She needs to believe it."

"Some professional advice," Jill said. "Suzy needs to express her fears. She needs to share them with you. Don't feel like you have to keep cheering her up."

I thought about how hard I had been trying to think, act and feel positive, and how unsuccessful I had been. I was grateful for Jill's observation.

Burton narrowed his eyes and slowly nodded. "I get it," he said.

Jill had trained with medical intuitive Carolyn Myss, who analyzes people and their illnesses through archetypes. She left me with a copy of Myss' recent book, *Sacred Contracts*. I put my feet up on the swing and began to read. Within a few pages, my stomach again became an over-inflated tire. The book made me feel as though I had given myself cancer, and if I didn't change my attitude, I might not beat it.

Jill had told me to befriend myself. That, I decided, meant refusing to read on.

I put the book onto a shelf and, instead, picked up my journal.

> *My Fears.*
> *Not being around to watch my children thrive.*
> *Missing the chance to develop the closeness with my granddaughter that I enjoyed with my grandmother.*
> *Burton's finding another life companion ...*

Within five minutes, my list numbered fifteen. ...

Later, I read my list to Burton. He sat and he listened. Without a word, he put his arms around me.

Later still, I picked up my journal again. ...

> *Gifts of This Experience*

(It took restraint not to write: nightmare).

> *My family has really rallied around me.*
> *Burton has been astonishing in his devotion and support.*
> *I have taken the time to revel in little Alexis.*
> *I'm dragging. Napping twice a day. This could be the last time I feel well for a while. I need to enjoy it, to stay in the moment. Easier said ...*

For many years, our family had taken holiday-card photos. When the boys were young, it was a challenge to get them to comb their hair, to hold still and smile and not to push each other out of the frame. As they grew older, the challenge graduated to agreeing on a time and date and setting. Daughters-in-law added the challenge of good hair days. Now there was a new generation to include, and the hope of finding a photo in which baby Alexis faced the camera and looked happy.

Our sons always accused me of picking the photo with the best picture of me. They were wrong. Like any sensible mother-in-law, I picked the image with the best shot of my daughters-in-law. We had not yet discovered Photoshop which in the future would let us move faces from one picture to another, allowing everyone to look their best, and fostering peace in the family.

By the time everyone agreed to show up for the annual photo, it was usually near December, and I had to rush to get cards printed, addressed and sent in time. In early August, four days before my surgery, the whole family was up north. Our sons made the remarkable suggestion that we shoot our holiday-card family photo. Nobody mentioned the reason for such efficiency.

The family gathered at the inland lake near our home and sat on or knelt around a log by the campfire pit. The sun shone. David didn't make horn fingers behind Andy's head. Andy didn't stand on his tiptoes to appear taller than David. Everyone smiled on cue and asked to be in a separate photo with me. I smiled, too, and held my chin high.

After, I fled to the farmhouse, curled up on the small window seat in my closet, and wept.

When you're making life or death decisions, you seek lots of advice. Lots of advice can confuse you. Every night I slept with the Wisdom Stone Marilyn had given me. Still I was confused. Burton was, too.

Our visit to Sloan-Kettering in New York had cost us ten more days. It unnerved me to think an alien force had gained extra time to spread its tentacles inside me, but Burton wanted to be as sure as he could about the treatment we pursued. He was relieved when Dr. Barakat, the chief gynecologist, spoke highly of Dr. Malone and agreed with his diagnosis and approach. I was too twisted with worry to share much relief.

David checked with a well-respected, retired Detroit gynecologist, Dr. Sherman. He recommended I undergo a radical or Wertheim hysterectomy. Dr. Malone disagreed. "The less you do, the less harm you might cause," he said. A radical approach could result in greater blood loss and subsequent bladder and rectal dysfunction. For yet another opinion, my sister called an oncologist friend. He agreed with Dr. Malone.

As the date for my surgery neared, Anne came in from California. I was glad to see my sister. We hadn't been together for three months. We looked alike, though Anne got the better hair and singing ability. Unlike me, Anne saw every glass as half full. Her perpetual optimism could be irritating, especially when the glass involved was mine. She sat at the foot of my bed, rubbing my feet. A foot rub is one of my favorite experiences. Anne knew just where to press. "Think good thoughts," she chirped. "Know that only good can come." As long as she continued pressuring the right spots, I let her chirp away.

When we were young, I regularly bounced my sister from my bedroom. Anne would prance around in my new kitten-heeled pumps. She butted in when I hung out with friends. She borrowed my beloved LP of *West Side Story* or helped herself to a piece of quartz or hematite from my mineral collection. I was always preparing for greatness—either to become a Broadway star, despite the fact I had no discernible musical talent, or to someday make history finding a significant fossil or meteorite. I had no time for my sister's peskiness.

The instant I left home for Ann Arbor, my sister turned into a delightful human being. Ever since, I have loved her company. As an adult, for a few years Anne lived with her family in nearby Birmingham. She taught at Brookside, a private elementary school, where she organized fourth graders into creating and performing charming, original musical plays. At the end of every school year, she composed and sang a song in which she named each student in her class. I was so proud the year she won the Outstanding Teacher award. Soon after, I sobbed through her going-away party just days before she and her family moved across country to Santa Barbara.

Anne had lived in California for almost fifteen years. I had last seen her in May when we shared a suite at Mii amo in Sedona, Arizona. Anne and a few close girlfriends had joined me for three days to celebrate my sixtieth birthday at the luxury spa tucked among red rock mountains. We enjoyed massages and facials. We stretched in yoga class and stepped and kicked with an exercise instructor. With a sore groin, I'd kept up the best I could. We had our fortunes told, and mine contained no mention of any health challenge. When I blew out the candles on my cake, I wished, as usual, for long, fruitful, healthy lives and relationships for my family and friends.

In Sedona, a guide escorted some of us through a vortex, one of several powerful energy sources in the area. He showed us how to create a medicine wheel. We clambered down to a dry river bed, picked up stones the size of small melons and carried them back to higher ground. We placed our stones on the dry, pale red earth in the shape of a circle with a cross inside. The cross pointed north, south, east and west.

We walked around the wheel and stopped when we felt a surge of energy. I circled three times. Each time I reached the western axis, my skin tingled. When we all found points we preferred, we sat on the ground at those points.

"Native Americans use the medicine wheel as a divining tool," our guide said. He walked around us, explaining the points on the wheel. Stopping behind me, he said something that made me shiver. "Try to give up your desire to control events. Trust that the universe will support you."

At the time, I thought the guide was talking about our upcoming *Oprah* appearance, three days away. During the entire process of writing my first book, I worried that discussing our problems so publicly could hurt my marriage, my family and our business. Such a giant forum as Oprah's, with seven million viewers, made me worry even more. The guide's words at the medicine wheel had helped give me courage.

Now, three months later, two days from surgery and more afraid than ever, I remembered the message I received that day in Arizona. It had, I realized, an even deeper significance.

I wrote a letter to Alexis, who was too young to read it, and to my future descendants. Andy wrote a letter to me. He described how he appreciated my cheering him on at baseball and football games, how he'd gotten his love of art and language and travel from me. Andy knew I had been trying to give up refined sugar, which fueled cancer cells, according to some nutritionists. He also knew my doctor had advised me to avoid solid foods for at least two days before surgery. Andy prepared a serving dish of sugar-free gelatin flavored with blueberry extract. "I figured out how to make Jell-O," he said with pride. I relished every bite. Of my two sons, Andy had been more disturbed by *Back from Betrayal*. He was a private young man whose father was his hero. The letter and the Jell-O showed me that while he may not have appreciated what I wrote, he supported and loved me anyway.

David had been less troubled by my book. His response at the time: "Whatever." Now our older son called with additional encouragement.

"We have to trust that God knows what He's doing, Mom, and we have to take the ride," David said. "I'll be with you every inch of the way. I won't let you quit. Leave the technical side to Dad and me and the doctors. You just get ready to fight. If God takes you to it, God will take you through it."

"That's beautiful," I said. "What sage said that?"

"Cedrick Ervin."

"Who's Cedrick Ervin?"

"A back-up tailback for the Detroit Lions."

For my darling Alexis and any siblings or cousins you might have:

Here are some lessons I've learned in sixty years of living. May they serve you well.

Be yourself. Find your strengths and go with them. Do what you love and you'll excel.

Tune in to your inner knowing. As the Buddha said: Listen to others, but only believe what you know in your heart to be true.

Stay in the moment. Savor each experience—from a walk to a talk to a hug. (I preach better than I practice.)

An open heart brings more joy than a closed mind. Everything and everyone provides lessons.

Have faith in a Higher Power. Your grandfather's and my problems made me realize the peace that comes from trusting in God. We only get the bigger picture when we look back on all the events that brought us where we are.

Be a fighter. Fight for yourself, your family, your beliefs. Tomorrow I face a painful surgery, frightening news and months of debilitating treatment. I'll fight my hardest to get through all of it so your grandfather and I can come to know you better and cheer you through your challenges.

Celebrate yourself and your family. Continue to appreciate your amazing parents. You have inherited an awesome legacy. Engage it. Enjoy it.

All my love,

Your adoring Gigi

I was grateful to survive two days without solid food and without a headache. My surgery took place on August 23rd, almost a month after cancer was first suspected. The operation, the less-aggressive approach Dr. Malone preferred, took two and a half hours. After, my surgeon visited my room. I was still groggy, but I remember his most important words. "No surprises," he said. "The operation was an A-plus."

My tummy felt tender but not terribly sore. The left side of my chest was tender, too, from a chemo port, inserted during surgery. Burton held my arm as I hobbled to the nurses' station on the day of surgery. I managed without Xanax for the first time in weeks.

When I was more coherent, Dr. Malone returned to share the pathology findings. I had a high-grade endometrial (uterine) adenocarcinoma. It penetrated both ovaries, the wall of my uterus and my pelvis. It was type one (not hormone-receptive), grade three (poorly-differentiated). Thankfully, it had not spread to my abdomen.

Three days after surgery, the epidural to control pain was removed. I received intravenous Dilaudid. My dressings were changed. I made myself look. I discovered the incision below my navel had been neither stapled nor sewn, but glued. I marveled that two sides of my tummy were stuck together without visible support and should heal in a neat vertical line. I hoped I'd live long enough for it to matter.

Four days after surgery I felt sluggish and discouraged. I berated myself over and over. How could I have been so naive as to think having intercourse could cause a groin pull? If only I had listened to my body, paid attention, seen a doctor sooner, the cancer might not have spread. I beat myself up with if onlys. And I beat myself up for beating myself up. Wondering if Vicodin and Darvocet were worsening my depression, I substituted Extra Strength Tylenol.

Returning home, I poked through a bottom drawer and found some baggy, nylon underpants. Three years before, in the wake of our marriage crisis, Brenda had talked me into buying sexier, new bikini panties. Although she counseled me to throw out the old ones, I had hung on to them. Now, grateful for my frugality, I realized my rejects put less pressure on my sore tummy. I snipped open the elastic legs for added comfort. Sex appeal was the least of my concerns.

Until the seventeenth century, hysteria was thought to be a medical condition caused by disturbances of the uterus. The Greek derivation of the word uterus is *hustera*. Plato believed the uterus was a separate spirit, an animal-part of a woman that wanted to become pregnant and created hysteria when it didn't. Hippocrates thought female hysteria came from the irregular movement of blood to the brain from the uterus. As for me, having lost my uterus, I was too lethargic for hysteria.

Five days after surgery, I felt lower than dust under a rug.

The most depressed I've ever felt. I want to be cheerful for Burton and my family and friends and especially for myself. I know it's illogical, but I feel guilty to have gotten sick and guilty for worrying people. The pain in my stomach has never been as bad as the pain in my heart. When I was home with viral pneumonia as a child, Mom told me: "It's darkest before the dawn." God, please let the dawn come soon.

CHAPTER 6

A Long Way from Kickboxing

Courage doesn't always roar. Sometimes courage is the little voice at the end of the day that says, "I'll try again."

—Mary Anne Radmacher-Hershey

BARBARA AND I met in the late sixties when I interviewed her for *Women's Wear Daily*. An executive with Federal's, Barbara raved about the creative programs the department store had begun and the charm school she had started and about how business was improving. Despite her zeal, the chain closed a few years later. Barbara went on to found and run a successful retail ad agency. As a consultant to Kmart, she discovered a little known east-coast society caterer who had published a cookbook. She recommended her to Kmart as a way to build their home accessories department. That little-known caterer was Martha Stewart.

Barbara and her husband had moved to Florida several years before to lessen the stress in their lives. Barbara had recovered from a supposedly incurable autoimmune disease and then from breast cancer. Some twenty years later, she was still healthy. Like my sister, she remained one of the most upbeat people I knew.

"You aren't physically sick," Barbara said. "You had something in your body. It's out now. This is an inconvenience. Our brains have the power to heal us. Think good thoughts."

Sitting next to Barbara in our library, fingering the cinnabar chenille sofa, I tried to think up something more cheerful than the inconvenience of my imminent demise and the fact that I had to pee for the twentieth time that day. I knew my friend meant well, but now, as if I didn't have enough to worry about, I worried about my inability to match Barbara's cheerfulness. If my brain could heal me, could it also make me sicker? Jill told me to face my fears; Barbara said forget about them. This was very confusing.

"I suck at positive thinking."

Barbara gave me the sort of look a parent gives a child who has fallen and skinned her knee. "Depression is something we can work on. Focus on your ability to make yourself better. Develop things to look forward to. My advice is: Make plans. You can always break them. Make them."

Before she left, Barbara gave me a book. "I bought it for the title," she said.

The name of the book: *Courage.*

Chemo class. Karmanos Patient Library. Burton and I watched a depressing video. Call the doctor if your port looks different, the video said. If your urine changes. If you start to cough or get chills. If you bleed from any orifice; have nausea, diarrhea or vomiting for more than twenty-four hours. Develop white spots in your mouth. Other possible side effects: fatigue, decreased red and/or white blood cells, hair loss, numbness in your hands and feet.

After, a nurse talked about maintaining my weight, about the aversion I might feel to the smell of meat. She advised grazing all day, drinking enough fluids to keep my kidneys pumping. And avoiding caffeine and black pepper (which retains bacteria), sticking to cooked vegetables when white cell counts drop, rinsing my mouth with salt water to help prevent sores.

Home later, my heart racing, I swallowed one Zoloft, then another. The two pills left me so tired that I put the rest back in a cupboard. Worn out from the antidepressant and from diarrhea, I started to cry. Again.

"What are you thinking?" Burton asked.

"I'm afraid of the next few months." I admitted something I hadn't had the nerve to say. "I'm afraid I'll lose you."

He cocked his head and raised his eyebrows. "You've got to be kidding. We started out with a couple of deuces. We're beginning to get some aces. We're starting chemotherapy. You're in better shape than most. You practice good nutrition. As for losing me? Forget it. I'm hooked forever. I'm in the boat. You'll never get rid of me." He put his baby finger into his mouth and pulled on his cheek.

"We have so much to live for," he said. "You are a healthy, beautiful woman."

I refrained from snorting. Ashen skin, no make-up, old-lady panties and straggly hair on its way out of town did not destine me for *People's* 50 Most Beautiful. But, bless my husband if he perceived some sort of inner beauty.

Burton put his hands on my shoulders and looked into my eyes. I've always had a weakness for Burton's eyes. The top lids are hooded; the irises, flecked with bits of green and brown.

"The difference between feeling good and feeling shitty is between your ears. No different than your golf game. Besides, you have to stay alive. I still expect you to write my eulogy."

That night I awoke from a dream. I was always surprised to wake up from a dream. It meant I had fallen asleep. For many years I had suffered from insomnia, a problem worsened by menopause, my diagnosis and my doctor's taking me off hormones. I dreamt Burton and I were on vacation in a strange city. I got lost and boarded a bus. I couldn't pay the fare because I didn't have my purse, but the driver drove me around searching for the house where we were staying. Eventually, he gave up and dropped me off. A woman passing by gave me money to call Burton. The phone was busy. A man stopped his car to offer directions.

Usually, on waking from a troubling dream, I felt relief. Now I woke up feeling afraid. My life had become a Maurice Sendak forest of wild things. My dream was better than my reality. Then I realized what the dream was really about. Despite my lack of control over what was happening, people kept helping me. And in the unfamiliar, chaotic land of cancer, I needed them all.

In September, the Ryder Cup took place at Oakland Hills Country Club where I had played (read: attempted to play) a few weeks before. The previous spring, Burton and I had attended the Masters Tournament in Augusta. We savored pimento and cream cheese sandwiches and admired mounds of pink-flowering azaleas. I ignored my sore groin as we marched from fairway to fairway and watched Phil Mickelson win his first Masters and Arnie Palmer play his last. I had come home and told friends Arnie Palmer had talked to me. "What did he say?" they asked. "He yelled 'fore!'" Glibness had since abandoned me. I wondered how I had ever come up with such a clever remark.

There was great excitement in Detroit over the Ryder Cup coming to town. Suburban streets were cordoned off; nearby houses rented for many thousands of dollars. Tiger Woods, who at that point still retained godlike stature, was playing. Normally, the journalist and the golfer in me would have wanted to be part of the action. If there were a movie or a restaurant or a blockbuster exhibit everyone was talking about or if the Red Wings or Pistons were in play-offs, I wanted to watch or attend, and the sooner the better. I got a rush from being part of the newest, biggest, most exciting whatever. Now, not only was I too enervated to attend the Ryder Cup, I didn't care about it.

I did care that Burton take a break from worrying about me. Since my diagnosis, he had rarely left my side. A friend invited him to play golf. I insisted he go. When he returned, he told me that on one hole he had missed a birdie putt. Whenever we played golf together and he scored a birdie, I sang a refrain from "Rockin' Robin."

"I didn't really try," he said. "My heart wasn't in it. You weren't there to sing."

Days later, up north, I again encouraged Burton to play golf. I was sitting on our porch swing, reading, when the phone rang. It was Burton, on his cell phone, calling from the 14th green at Belvedere.

"I just sunk a twenty-foot putt for a birdie," he said. "Sing."

My voice croaked. But I sang.

Sara, a college student, practiced Yoga and had massage training. Burton hired her to help during afternoons while I recovered from surgery and underwent chemo. As she rubbed my grateful feet, I asked if she had a favorite prayer.

"A poem, actually. 'Footprints in the Sand.'" She pressed deep into my right arch. "A woman falls asleep and dreams of a beach. She sees footprints in the sand and realizes they represent her life. Mostly there are two sets of prints. She sees them as God's and hers. She thinks back on her life. When times were toughest, she sees only one set of prints. In her dream she asks God why He deserted her when she needed Him most."

"And?"

"God replies, 'Those weren't the times I deserted you. Those were the times I carried you.'"

Later, Sara drove me to the dentist. Since chemo can cause bleeding, patients are advised to see a dentist before treatment. I took along my new book, *Courage*. Waiting for the dentist, I leafed through. The book contained thoughts and stories on courageous women. I read a few paragraphs of a passage called "Embracing Faith." The dentist showed up and fixed a crumbled filling in a bottom front tooth.

As Sara drove me home, I flipped to the passage I had skimmed in the dentist's chair and read it to her. Then I noticed the story that followed. It told of Eva, whose first child was born with cerebral palsy and who suffered other hardships, including poverty and depression. For solace, Eva turned to a poem by a poet named Mary Stevenson. It hung on her living room wall. The poem was reprinted in the book.

Reading the title, I caught my breath. Eva's favorite poem: "Footprints in the Sand."

Your first official appointment after surgery is a scary time. To walk into an examining room knowing you have passed a major hurdle is heartening. But you also know the news you will hear will determine your subsequent treatment and chances of recovery.

Burton was anxious, too. Instead of his usual golf shirt and Brooks Brothers navy sweater, he wore a sport jacket and tie. When Dr. Malone walked into the examining room, Burton stood up and shook his hand. "I wore this tie," he said, "to show my respect for you."

Dr. Malone smiled and touched the patterned blue knot at his throat. "I always wear a tie," he said. "Out of respect for my patients."

Dr. Malone approved of how my incision was healing. I had been slathering on antibiotic ointment; the redness and swelling had diminished.

I was nervous to hear what my physician had learned about the lymph nodes he had removed during surgery. Lymph nodes are a delivery system. If cancer showed up in my lymph nodes, there was a greater chance it would spread elsewhere.

"The surgery to remove your ovaries and uterus got rid of ninety to ninety-five percent of the malignant cells in your body," Dr. Malone said. "Your lymph nodes were clear."

I exhaled with relief. Burton squeezed my hand. I looked at him, handsome in his navy jacket and red tie, a look he seldom wore since he retired about five years before. His eyes glistened.

"The tumors in your ovaries were necrotic, or nearly dead, from lack of blood supply," Dr. Malone said. "The cancer was either clear-cell or endometrial. Some doctors would argue they're the same. In either case, the treatment is the same.

"What about my thyroid?"

"That cancer may be unrelated or may have spread through your bloodstream. For now, I'd advise leaving it alone. It will function as a marker of how well chemotherapy is working."

Dr. Malone said he wanted to repeat the MRI of my brain. "The spots we saw earlier may indicate another metastasis."

"Brain cancer?" I groaned. That was a worry even I hadn't thought of. My heart pounded. I longed for a Xanax.

"Or they might just have come from the way you laid on the table."

"What are the symptoms of brain cancer?"

"Stumbling."

"I'm a klutz."

"Forgetfulness."

"No more than usual."

"Headaches."

I shook my head and knocked on it.

My chemo regimen would consist of carboplatin and Taxol, typical for uterine-, ovarian- and breast-cancer patients, Dr. Malone said. I also needed radiation to my pelvis. Without it, my lesions could grow larger and destabilize the bone. I would receive six rounds of chemo, one every three weeks. Chemo would begin two weeks after surgery. Radiation, five days/week for six-and-a-half weeks, would start two weeks after my first chemo. For several weeks, I'd receive chemo and radiation concurrently.

"Aggressive cancer requires aggressive treatment," Dr. Malone said. "We consider you young and healthy enough to handle it."

Young? Sixty and falling apart. Healthy? Even though my doctor had seen me from the bottom up and inside out, healthy was a stretch.

"There's a good chance you'll make it through all the treatment," Dr. Malone said. "We're shooting for a cure."

I am a lover of words. They connect us to friends; they warn us of danger; they inform and enlighten and entertain us. They introduce us to other worlds. I heard a lot of medical terms during my diagnosis and treatment. Some were terrifying; some, confusing. I heard encouraging words as well. Young was good. Healthy was better yet. But none was as uplifting as that single word, the word that for me evoked sunny days and rippling water and the promise of hope. The single word: cure.

"Close your eyes and relax," Rebekka said.

I had experienced energy work once before. Two years before, I had visited the Canyon Ranch Spa in Arizona with my girlfriend Sandy who owned a time share there. That week I was feeling especially vulnerable. Burton and I had been working to heal our marriage for about three years. Sandy's boyfriend, Charley, had left a sweet message on the phone in our room. Burton's voice had sounded distant, and that was all I needed for my insecurities to flare. At the spa I went for long walks, danced to African drumbeats in class, enjoyed a facial and a Swedish massage, but still I felt tense. I wanted to cry, but my tears were stuck like iron particles in a faucet.

Sandy recommended an energy massage. "It's not like a regular massage," she advised. I signed up.

Running her hands lightly up and down my body, my energy therapist said, "Your female organs seemed blocked. How's your relationship?"

Realizing what my body had revealed, I felt a sob push past my clogged chest. I bawled through the rest of the treatment. After, my therapist led me to a quiet room to compose myself. I didn't need to compose. I felt better than I had in days.

Now I lay on Rebekka's portable table under a blanket in the small sitting room just off our bedroom. Rebekka held her hands above me and moved them up and down my body, avoiding any pressure on my sore tummy. I peeked through half-closed eyes. Rebekka had long, graying brown hair caught in a band at her neck and gentle, watery-blue eyes. She wore a patterned, shapeless nurse's top. Occasionally her hands stopped and pressed lightly. Balancing my energy, she said.

"I sense weakness in two of your chakras." Chakra is Sanskrit for wheel or turning point, she explained. Our bodies have seven major chakras, or life-energy centers, also called *prana* or *shakti* or *qi*. Chakras are a concept from traditional Indian medicine.

She touched my hips. "The pelvic area, or second chakra, concerns our family of origin and other tribes. Tribes maintain rules to survive. They send strong messages about being a good wife, daughter and mother."

She touched my throat. "The fifth chakra involves communication. How we speak our truth, how we're heard, how we talk to ourselves. You seem challenged in both areas."

When I was first diagnosed, I felt angry with my body for betraying me. Now I felt sad. Cancer had invaded my female organs and my thyroid. Without my telling her, Rebekka had sensed both problems. My body had supported me for sixty years in spite of the emotional strain I put it through. Worrying about and rebuilding my marriage. Writing and publishing a difficult memoir. Feeling responsible for my mother's well-being.

A decade earlier, at seventy, Mom was diagnosed with Parkinson's Disease. She began taking L-DOPA and seemed to fare well. She continued to play bridge, to golf and garden. Months later, for no clear reason, Mom's big toe turned into a hammer-toe and a monkey toe. It stuck up and stuck out. She decided to have surgery. "Foot surgery is a big deal," I warned. She said, "Don't try to scare me. I don't want to wear old-lady shoes for the rest of my life." And so I accompanied her to see the highly-recommended doctor she chose and to the hospital for surgery.

Mom emerged with a pin in her left big toe. Her bulky cast pointed down and to the right. She complained about it. Days later, I took her back to the doctor. He had been unable to bend Mom's ankle after surgery, he said, and was forced to cast it the way he did. He removed the cast and tried to bend her left foot.

It was frozen in a toe-down, turned-in position. The doctor recast it the same way as before.

After the cast came off, Mom's foot resembled a club foot. Her surgeon could not explain the complication; nor could any other doctor. Mom was forced to hobble, putting pressure on her ankle. Soon, she tripped over her walker and broke her leg. She lay, recovering, in a convalescent home for several weeks wearing a full-leg cast.

Fearing Mom would never walk again (she never did), Anne and I agreed we could not let her move back to the Birmingham apartment she loved. She was the only occupant of the small, three-story building aside from the landlady upstairs. We decided to move her to a senior citizen complex. We found a smaller, two-bedroom apartment at The Trowbridge in Southfield, near my home. At seventy-one, Mom was chronologically young for such a residence. But, there were nurses available. She could make friends, eat meals, get her hair done, play bridge, listen to lectures—all things she enjoyed. She could go on outings in a wheelchair-equipped van. There was a bedroom for the full-time aide she now required. Mom opposed the move. Since none of us had a better idea, we proceeded. My friend and interior designer, Rick, helped Anne and me move Mom's possessions. We hung pictures and arranged antiques and recreated her previous apartment as closely as we could. We bought her an electric wheelchair so she could get around on her own.

Mom couldn't, or wouldn't, adjust. She had her hair done downstairs and ate dinner with her aide in the dining room for a couple of months. After those first attempts, she would not leave her apartment. No encouragement on Anne's and my part would budge her. Her blonde bouffant turned gray and straight. Her nails grew long enough to bend under until her aide clipped them. She had meals delivered upstairs. She sat in the apartment day after day, year after year, watching TV, reading, sometimes doing a word puzzle in the local paper. She waited for calls from Anne and me and took notes on what we said. The next day she asked us about the party or meeting we had mentioned earlier. She collected the notes on our conversations in a pile on the dining table and would not let us throw them out. It was as though her life had shrunk down to that little stack of notepaper. She discouraged her old friends from calling, protesting, "I don't have anything to say." She folded in on herself the way her foot folded in on her leg.

A few years before, after praying for release from my sense of responsibility for my mother, I stopped worrying so much about her. I cut down my frequent visits to see her and also cut down the drinking which had helped me escape her problems. I focused more on my life and less on hers. But, I felt guilty for not being more attentive, for not being what I viewed as a better daughter.

I said to Rebekka, "I guess I gave myself more than I could handle."

Rebekka's hands continued to glide and alight like sunbeams. "Ask your higher self for help," she said. "Be open for a miracle."

Adjusting her fluffy brown wig with her fingers, Patsy said, "I used to be into beauty. A few months before my first diagnosis, I had some spider veins and facial hair removed. All of a sudden, I found myself in chemo without a hair on my body. I went from looking swell to looking like hell. Didn't God have the last laugh?"

Patsy Ramsey and her husband, John, joined us for lunch on the porch of our farmhouse. In the past two years, Patsy had suffered two recurrences of ovarian cancer. Still, she came to the farmhouse to give me support. Cancer is a club no one wants to join, but those who do look out for each other.

"You were into beauty, alright. Even with vegetables," I said.

Eight years earlier, four months before her daughter was murdered, Patsy and six-year-old JonBenét visited our farm to pick from our vegetable garden. Patsy's cancer had not yet returned. Her cheeks were pink; her hair, once again dark and shiny. She looked like an older version of the Miss America contestant she had once been.

A zucchini about three feet long sat on our white, laminate kitchen counter.

Patsy said, "That would win first prize at the County Fair."

"Probably would," I said.

"Will you enter it?"

"Probably not."

I avoided competition. As a teen I made one exception. I entered the *Seventeen Magazine* guest-editor competition and advanced to the semi-finals. But hearing that several hundred other young women did too, I pulled out. I knew I lacked the time and will to work hard enough to win. Whether I had the talent, I would never know. There was safety in not knowing. We make choices, and we pay for them. If I didn't give all my energy to one area, I had energy left over for others. I could be good enough. I could be the mother who accompanied her kids on Halloween but clad them in store-bought costumes, who showed up at their baseball games with cookies from the market. The wife who was available to travel with her husband but maintained a part-time career. I have always been a fan of moderation. *Back from Betrayal* was a rare exception. I gave it everything I had. That's one reason I remained proud of it.

Patsy left our farmhouse that afternoon cradling a zucchini the size of a three-month-old baby; JonBenét carried a bag of broccoli and beans. Days later, Burton and I stopped at the fair in Petoskey. In the produce section we found our zucchini, entered in our names and those of Patsy and JonBenét. It was oiled to a sheen, nested on a red-and-white checkered cloth napkin in the perfect oval wicker basket. Beside it lay a blue ribbon. Our zucchini, the beauty queen of the produce pageant.

Eight years later, Patsy and John and Burton and I had been through a lot. Patsy knew her odds for living much longer weren't good. Still she managed to grin. "I told you that zucchini was a star," she said.

I thanked Patsy for suggesting I have a port inserted during my surgery. "My chest still feels sore."

"Give it time." Hers had gotten her through two recent rounds of chemo, she said. She pulled down the neck of her blue t-shirt to show me the bump in her chest. She patted it with her hand. "It's more comfortable than my wig, actually. But I'm grateful for both of them."

Patsy didn't seem cowed by the fear that had crippled me. I said, "With everything you've been through, I feel like such a baby. But I'm on the verge of crying all the time. How do you stay so positive?"

"My motto is: Fiddledeedee. I'll worry tomorrow," she said and batted her big, blue eyes. "That's from the new, revised Southern-version of the Bible."

"I mean seriously?"

"Seriously?" She lifted her palms up. "The same way I got through losing my only daughter. My faith. I believe I'll see Jon-Benét again."

I shook my head. "You're amazing."

"People are like precious metal. We start out as rock. It takes pressure and heat to shape a rock into a thing of beauty. God refines us by fire. He loves us too much to leave us as rocks."

When Patsy and John were about to leave, this three-time cancer survivor and bereaved parent gave me another demonstration of her resilience. She stopped at the door and turned to me.

"You'll feel better when you begin treatment," she said. "That's when you start to kick ass." She jogged in place, lifting her knees high and punching her fists in the air.

As the Ramseys' car receded down the dirt road, Burton and I stood on the porch watching dust rise. Burton put his arm around me.

"I wish my faith was that strong," I said. "I'm a long way from kickboxing."

CHAPTER 7

Heaven Can Wait

Most emotions are responses to perception—what you think is true about a given situation. If your perception is false, then your emotional response to it will be false, too.

—William Paul Young, *The Shack*

THE WEISBERG CENTER, where I would soon begin radiation, was a stone and wood building that resembled a contemporary Western ski lodge. Inside, water ran down a two-story green-tiled wall in the foyer. Hallways were hung with black-and-white photos of Cranbrook in nearby Bloomfield Hills, shot by renowned photographer, Balthazar Korab, with whom I had once shared a column in the *Detroit News*. I found, styled and wrote about decorating vignettes. Digi (Korab's nickname) photographed them. Cranbrook was a private educational campus begun in the 1920s by newspaper publisher George Booth and designed by famed architect Eliel Saarinen. Cranbrook Academy of Art alumni included legendary design names like Knoll and Eames. My sister and I had attended Kingswood, the girls' school at Cranbrook; Andy had attended the boys' school. (The schools have since merged.) As an adult, Anne taught at Brookside, the elementary school.

On my first visit, the Weisberg Center seemed as though it would be a striking setting for a cocktail party. But the cocktails dispensed in the back came in I.V. tubes, not martini glasses.

We met with Katherine, the staff psychologist. "How are you doing emotionally?" she asked.

"Not well."

"The biggest mistake couples make is trying to protect each other's feelings," she said. "It's okay to have a meltdown together."

Burton and I had heard this advice before. We couldn't hear it often enough.

In the lobby, I had noticed a sign on the reception desk. A support group for patients with women's cancers was in progress.

"Tell me about the group," I said.

"These gals have been together for several months. They're real fighters. And a big help to each other. Would you like to sit in?"

I nodded. "It might be good to know people with similar problems."

Katherine escorted me down the hall, past display cases filled with art glass, and into a conference room. About ten women sat around a table. They looked up as we entered.

"Suzy is new here," Katherine said.

"Welcome," one said. She had thick brown hair. A wig, I guessed. "I'm Judy. Breast cancer. Fighting it on and off for five years."

"Carol," the woman beside her said. "Ovarian. Diagnosed six years ago."

As they took turns telling me their names and diseases, I sensed the grit of these women and their affection for each other. They welcomed me warmly, and my disease certainly qualified me to be here. Still, I felt uncomfortable.

Natalie was the last to introduce herself. She wore a turban. "Breast," she said. "Eight years. Spread to my lungs, but I'm still here." She patted her turban. "How about you?"

"Uterine," I said. "Seven weeks."

Natalie shook her head. "Welcome to the roller coaster."

"Thanks ... I think." I saw some nods, heard some humphs. "Please go on with your meeting."

"Okay," Carol said. "I couldn't wait to tell you all about this one. A few days ago, I received a present from a so-called friend, someone I've known for a long time. She sent me a book, *A Travel Guide to Heaven*." She shrugged her shoulders. "I guess she meant to do me a favor. I sure as hell don't want that book."

"Some people just don't get it," said a pretty young blonde. "Heaven may be a popular destination. But it can damn well wait."

"Yeah," Natalie said. "Not a lot of people rushing to Expedia checking out the airfare."

Carol smiled. "How should I respond?"

"Tell her to stick that book up her ass," Natalie said, to general laughter, clapping and pounding on the table.

"Second the motion," another said.

A woman sitting a few seats away wore a pink t-shirt reading Connie's Fun 'n Funds. "I'm still selling tickets for the picnic to raise money for my bone marrow transplant," she said. "It's a bargain. Ten bucks a ticket. All the fried chicken you can eat. Food's all donated. The picnic is this Sunday. I hope some of you can make it."

"Count me in, Connie," Natalie said.

"Me, too," another said.

A woman next to Connie had brown hair sprinkled with grey, pulled back on one side with a tortoise barrette. "You all know I live alone," she said. "I have no one to hold me or touch me. It is what it is. I don't stew about it. I didn't realize how much I missed human contact until the other day. I went to the park with my brother and his autistic son Jeremy. Jeremy came up and put his arms around me. I know he did it because he was thirsty. He was reaching for the water bottle in my fanny pack. But it felt so good to have someone hug me that I actually started to cry."

Connie rubbed her hand. I swallowed hard.

At the end of the meeting, I said goodbye to some of the women and handed Connie twenty dollars. "Give the tickets to someone who can use them," I said.

I walked back down the hall to the lobby feeling a mix of admiration and sadness for the women I had met. And guilt for feeling sorry for myself when others faced even tougher challenges.

Burton looked up from his *Crain's Detroit Business.*

"How was it?" he asked.

"Interesting," I said. "Nice women."

"Let's reward ourselves," Burton said. We walked to the T-Bird.

"Okay if I put the top down?"

"What the heck," I said. My moisturizer was SPF 15 and it was a glorious day and who knew how long I'd have to worry about my complexion anyway.

Driving on Orchard Lake Road that sunny afternoon, we passed a strip shopping center. Standing on the curb, someone was dressed as a bumblebee, holding a sign advertising a flower shop, waving people in.

Cancer makes you more sensitive. "He must be hot in that costume," I said.

Burton said, "It's a tough day for bumblebees."

At Yoz I ordered a honey-sweetened smoothie mixed with blueberries and strawberries. I am expert at rationalizing my food choices. Yogurt was healthier than ice cream; honey was healthier than sugar; and fresh fruit was fiber, vitamins and antioxidants. As we headed home, I sat in the car slurping my thick, cold drink, thinking about the meeting. I didn't have to host picnics to fund my medical care. I had a husband whose affections may have been challenged in recent years, but whose devotion since I got sick was unswerving. A husband who waited for me in lobbies and hugged me whenever I needed it. I had a loving family and friends. I have so much to be grateful for, I thought, and felt ashamed not to feel more grateful.

I admired the courage of the women I met that day. I saw the help and concern they provided each other. But I didn't have the energy for a new set of friends. If I did make a new friend, I didn't want the focus of our relationship to be illness. If I joined these gutsy, good-hearted women, I'd become involved in their lives. I'd worry about them, and I had enough to worry about. And my new friends might not all survive.

I didn't go back.

Driving on Northwestern Highway to Whole Foods or Bed Bath & Beyond, I had often passed the Weisberg Clinic. I was thinking about organic arugula or a new tablecloth. Never about the patients inside the building receiving radiation or chemo. Or the loved ones who waited for them. Or how worried they all must be. Sitting in the lobby, waiting to meet my newest doctor, I could think of nothing else. I bounced my foot and worried about what harm radiation would do to me, and about what cancer would do to me without it. Both of my hips were sore. I still had pain moving my left leg sideways. I had to be here.

A nurse showed us into an examining room. I fingered the paper on the table. Burton reminded me of what we'd heard about Dr. Forman. That he'd trained at Johns Hopkins. That he'd worked at Sloan-Kettering. That people called him brilliant.

Dr. Forman walked in, wearing a white lab coat. His sandy-brown hair had a trace of spike. Doctors used to be combed, grey and venerable, I thought. When did they get so young?

"A large, soft tissue tumor has eaten away the top of your left pelvic bone; a smaller one, the lower right part of your pelvic bone," Dr. Forman said.

"What's soft tissue?"

"Muscle. Ninety percent of your left pelvic bone has disappeared; sixty percent of your right."

I shuddered. "I knew things were bad. But not ninety percent bad."

"Both sides of your pelvic bone will regenerate once the cancer cells disappear. Chemotherapy should kill most of them.

Radiation will destroy any that resist chemo. I think we can get rid of the lesions completely."

"Completely?" I hoped I'd heard right.

He raised his eyebrows and nodded. "Completely."

"How do you know how much radiation to give me?"

"As much as is safe, and we hope it's enough."

"How long will it take for my pelvis to heal?"

"Once the tumor is destroyed, bones heal within weeks to months."

"Side effects?"

"Exhaustion. Diarrhea. Bone marrow loss. All possible. The more slowly we deliver radiation, the more we can safely give you and the fewer side effects you'll have."

Soon after, I hopped off the table.

Dr. Forman winced. "Take it easy," he said. "That left pelvic bone could crack. It's like a board infested with termites. Favor your right leg."

Another small room. Another examining table. I lay back as a technician poked my skin with a needle. One poke below each hipbone, above my crotch and above my forehead. She dabbed blue ink on the holes, creating permanent dots to help line me up with the radiation machine. However stylish tattoos had become in recent years, I hoped I'd never need another.

Still lying down, I rested my legs in a bed of warm foam. It cooled, creating a plastic mold to hold my legs in place during radiation.

Minutes later, I returned to the nearby imaging center for another CT scan of my pelvis. Dr. Forman would use it to map out my radiation plan. Radiation would begin two weeks after my first chemo. For a while, I'd receive chemo and radiation simultaneously—an aggressive approach for an aggressive disease.

I wish they could take my body and fix it, and put my spirit or soul or whatever makes me, me, on autopilot for the next few months, and wake me when this is over.

Chemotherapy. The word frightens. Every cancer is different. Every body is different. Every reaction is different. At three-week intervals we would drive south on the John Lodge Expressway to Karmanos Cancer Institute. Karmanos was then one of about thirty-five hospitals in the nation to merit a Comprehensive Cancer Center designation from the National Institute of Health (NIH). That designation indicated superior expertise in research, education and clinical trials. As distressed as I was, I appreciated the chance to receive first-rate medicine near home, close to family and friends who supplied steady hugs and encouragement.

Before my first chemo, I sat at Karmanos in the crowded waiting area of the blood lab. Soon I was called into a smaller room. A few chairs had arm rests; a counter held dozens of test tubes. A nurse punched a needle into my port, the rubber device under the skin on my chest, then drew some blood through the needle. The poke hurt, but after that chemicals could be injected without further discomfort.

We trudged through a door into the chemo ward. Burton carried my tote bags, bulging with a tape player, headphones, CDs, books, magazines, my journal and a squishy travel pillow. I brought lemon drops to counteract any possible bad taste from chemo (which didn't occur) and Jon's stuffed, brown Chemo Bear.

Bags knocking against his thighs, Burton said, "I feel like a pack mule."

Hallways were lined with small, private rooms, each furnished with a twin bed and a chair. Each room had a window overlooking the hall. Most were occupied. A nurse showed me to a room that was free. I climbed on the bed and propped Chemo Bear by my side. The nurse connected an I.V. tube to the needle in my chest.

For the first hour, steroids were delivered through my port to counteract chills, fever or hives that could occur as side effects of poisonous chemicals. For the next three hours, a brew of carboplatin and Taxol snaked through the clear plastic tube. The infusion pump emitted a steady tick, whirr, tick, whirr. Padded earphones did not muffle the sound. At first I found it annoying. Then, with steroid-induced inspiration, I changed my attitude. In time to the machine, I silently said thank you, thank you for modern medicine that could eliminate harmful invaders from my body and, God willing, make me well.

I read, rested, listened to affirmations, journaled about endless worries. Burton took a walk with a friend, a hospital official. I listened to songs on the iPod Andy gave me the night before. He recorded more than 100 of his favorite songs and mine.

In the fall of Andy's junior year, he and I took a two-week driving trip through New England to visit colleges. He brought along a tape of a singer I had never heard. I fell in love with Van Morrison's gravelly voice and rough-edged lyrics and with one song about a "gypsy soul." I played "Into the Mystic" over and over as we drove.

Lying in bed in a chemo ward, listening to the song again, I was back in central New Hampshire. It was 1991. Andy and I had parked our rental car and hiked over a wooded ridge and thrilled to see Squam Lake stretch out before us. Squam Lake was the setting for the movie *On Golden Pond*, a family favorite. Whenever Burton fished with David and Andy, they competed to see who could catch a fish the size of Walter, the film's elusive big trout.

Andy decided on Bowdoin College in Maine. After one semester, he transferred to the University of Michigan, my alma mater, thus ensuring yet another rivalry with his big brother, a senior at Michigan State. During college, Andy spent a semester studying in Spain and six weeks traveling around Eastern Europe by himself. When Andy was a little boy, I taught him how to check airport monitors on our trips. He learned to tell us our boarding gate and whether or not our plane was on time. Andy grew up with an independent streak and a love of travel. A gypsy soul.

Andy had magically transformed into a parent. He would one day take his daughter and maybe other children to visit colleges. I longed to attend Alexis' graduation.

A volunteer stopped by with a lunch cart. Ham and cheese on whole wheat tasted good. Time passed. A nurse removed the needle and sent us home with anti-nausea medications.

I had read Lance Armstrong's *It's Not about the Bike*. His description of the vomiting he endured from chemo was so frightening that I skipped most of that part. I was relieved not to experience anything so horrific. Dr. Malone had cautioned me to take Zofran early and to add Compazine if I needed more help. Stay ahead of the nausea, he advised. I did, and my stomach cooperated.

As anxious as I felt, my first chemo was not as bad as I had feared.

Within hours, the relief I felt from surviving my first chemo was replaced by another round of terror. To pull me through, I phoned the psychotherapist who helped me survive our marriage crisis. A few years ago, Jim had encouraged me to see that I could function on my own if I had to. I hoped he could help propel me through my latest trauma. He assured me I was strong and determined enough to get through a health crisis as well.

"Stay centered and focused," he said. "Trust yourself. Know you can handle whatever comes. Fear enters when we lose our faith."

My heart continued to pound; my lungs leaked air.

"I can't help feeling so afraid," I said.

"Of what?"

Worried to speak my fear out loud, I whispered, "Dying."

"Hmm," he said. "Let's talk about that. What would be so terrible about dying?"

Usually I am polite to a fault. Not wanting to hurt someone else's feelings often comes before taking care of my own. Especially when that someone else is a person whose authority and insight I respect. But cancer was teaching me to be gentler with myself.

Over the pounding of my heart, I heard myself say, "I know you mean to help, Jim. I'm not ready to think about dying. I'll call you back if I am." And I hung up.

Several weeks later, Burton and I were booked to speak to the Michigan chapter of the Imago marriage counselors association. I admired the insightful approach of this group who helped wounded couples heal their relationships. I read founder Harville Hendrix's book, *Getting the Love You Want*, when Burton and I were working through our problems. Before I got sick, I had contacted the organization to schedule a speaking engagement. When I heard back, I was already ill. Still, I wanted to proceed. If *Back from Betrayal* was going to be my last contribution to humanity, I wanted to give it my best effort. Imago therapists could recommend my book to clients struggling with their own marriages, readers I hoped to reach. Chemo knocks you flat when first delivered. It takes several days to regain some strength. I arranged our talk to take place the night before my third chemo, timing that would maximize my energy.

Jim was in the audience that night. Before Burton and I spoke, he came up to me. "I want to apologize for our last conversation," he said. "I was out of line. I hope you'll forgive me."

"You were," I said. "And I do."

Back at the Weisberg Center, I passed a photograph of Swedish-born sculptor Carl Milles' Orpheus Fountain, one of dozens of bronzes at Cranbrook, and one I had admired often, in person. I guessed the serene photographs lining the hall were meant to distract patients from the less-than-serene process they were here to undergo. In a small changing room, I hung my sweat pants in a closet and slipped on a cotton gown. Two weeks had passed since my first chemo. I took a chair in the waiting room and flipped through a magazine, trying to get my mind off one of the last times I saw my father. It was nearly thirty years before. He had undergone radiation for colon cancer. His flesh had been so burned that a foul odor emanated from his wound. He died not long after.

Denise, a technician with a friendly smile and many small pins on the lapel of her white coat, greeted Burton and me. She showed us the radiation control room. With TV monitors and computer keyboards, it looked like it belonged at an airport.

A table in the center of the treatment room had a long glass top. A monitor sat above it. Also suspended from the ceiling was a machine about two feet square with a projecting cone. I eyed it with dread. Denise spread a white cotton sheet on the table and I lay down. Producing the mold made earlier, Denise slid it under my legs. My limbs trembled. Denise covered me with a sheet.

The radiation machine would rotate around me, Denise said. It would stop at designated points to deliver a beam for several seconds and then move on. I would hear a hum but wouldn't feel anything. I must lie very still.

Denise left the room. A heavy metal door clunked shut. The machine behaved as Denise described. Several minutes later, she returned and lowered the table. I eased myself down. Denise was right. I didn't feel a thing.

For the first few days, radiation was mostly a chance to lie still, pray and listen to Rod Stewart or Ella Fitzgerald sing. I liked Ella's spunky delivery of "Mack the Knife." A fitting touch of irony.

A few days into radiation, Dr. Forman examined me. At that point, the worst part of the experience was the embarrassment of having an attractive, younger doctor inspect and then discuss my labia and anus. They were turning red, he said, receiving more radiation than he liked. He would adjust the beam to minimize external damage.

Embarrassment would become the least of my radiation woes.

Our house in Franklin was quiet. Outside, a truck rumbled down the rutted, dirt road. I again lay beneath a blanket on

Rebekka's massage table. Rebekka moved her hands above me. I longed for pressure, for someone to push deep into my tense muscles, but this was energy therapy, not a deep tissue massage.

For several days I had felt like crying. My tears were dammed up, as they had once been at Canyon Ranch. Suddenly, unexpectedly, bad thoughts began spewing from my mouth. "I hate what's happening to my body. I hate feeling so tired. I hate the uncertainty. I hate not being in charge of my schedule. I hate the strain I've put on my family."

Rebekka's hands stopped to rest lightly and move on. "Our souls come to earth to learn lessons," she said softly. "Your soul volunteered for this challenge. Burton's and your sons' did, too."

"If I volunteered for this, I take it back," I wailed. "This is too hard."

Suddenly my legs, arms and torso started to shake. I trembled as though the temperature had dropped below freezing.

"Are you cold?" Rebekka asked, tucking another blanket around me.

Teeth chattering, I said, "I don't know." I was frightened. I had never lost control like this before.

Rebekka continued to press lightly at different points. In the calmest voice, she said, "This is good. You're getting rid of trapped negative energy. Go with it."

Still trembling, I feared I was having some kind of seizure.

Rebekka pressed lightly on my chest, my belly, my thighs. "Let it out."

After what seemed like forever, but may have five or ten minutes, my shaking subsided. My limbs sank into the table. A warm current flowed through me. I no longer needed to cry. For the first time in days, I felt my body relax.

"Visualize healing light filling up the spaces you emptied out," Rebekka said. Her hands flitted and alighted like butterflies. "To get through fear, you must stand nose to nose with it. Your shaking moved through you, and it lifted. That's the nature of everything energetic. If you have a bad day, have it. If you worry you'll get stuck in it, you give it power over you.

"People can stand by you, but they can't be in the ring with you. You are starving for your own love. No one else's love will fill that space. Hold every part of you as precious. Your body will get better if you appreciate it and recognize how far you've come.

"Every minute, ask yourself: What do I need now? You can handle each minute. Remember what Pogo said, 'I have seen the enemy, and it is me.' This experience is about finding your soul."

I opened my eyes and peered at Rebekka. She was surrounded by light.

Sitting up, I remembered something that happened the past winter, two months before my self-diagnosed groin pull. I awoke early one morning in Florida to find a transparent, three-dimensional man standing beside me. Startled, I called Burton's name, then looked at his side of the bed. He remained asleep. I turned back and the man was gone. My initial fear at this apparition dissolved. I decided he was some sort of guardian. My see-through man had returned four times since. He never lingered for more than a second, but I began to appreciate knowing he was there.

I told Rebekka about my transparent visitor. She smiled. "He'll help when panic overwhelms you. He's a healer."

Burton and I stopped in Royal Oak at Duggan's Irish Pub for lunch. Again feeling sorry for myself, I glanced at the next table. A young man sat in a wheelchair holding a fist near his pale, flat cheek. He mumbled unintelligible sounds to the grey-haired woman with him. She paid close attention. I assumed she was his mother. I remembered David's arm around me the night before, the arm with which he smashed a tennis serve or drew back an arrow. I thanked God again for healthy children. There were tougher problems than mine.

In the late fifties and sixties, before Burton and I met, we often frequented the Totem Pole, another restaurant in Royal Oak. "Buzzing the Pole" was a favorite activity for teens driving up and down Woodward Avenue in Mustangs and Chevys, radios blasting with Del Shannon singing "Runaway" or the Contours' "Do You Love Me." The popular drive-in restaurant served a Big Chief Burger, a hamburger topped with shredded lettuce, American cheese, sweet pickles and a savory sauce. After we met, Burton and I enjoyed Big Chief Burgers together, though the restaurant was no longer the hot spot of our youth. In 1972, our old hangout was replaced by a Burger King. We often took our little boys there but never with the same zeal we felt for its predecessor. The ingredients of the Totem Pole's secret sauce were never revealed. Many tried to figure out the recipe. I suspected it included curry powder, mayo and Worcestershire sauce, but no one knew for sure. What we did know was that we missed our Big Chief Burgers.

Several years after the Totem Pole closed, Burton and I visited a new restaurant not far from our house in Huntington Woods. Our waitress at Duggan's recommended the hamburgers.

She said, "Do you remember the Totem Pole?"

I said, "Don't tell me."

She raised her eyebrows and nodded.

"Prove it," I said.

She produced a sublime cheeseburger. Burton and I agreed: the piquant sauce was just as we remembered. My next weekly column in the *Detroit News* proclaimed the happy headline: **The Big Chief Burger is Back!**

Duggan's owner, Larry Payne, came up to our table, sat down and grinned at me. "You put us on the map," he said. "I still have a copy of that column."

I smiled, thinking about the power I once enjoyed. About how little power I had now.

"How are you?" Burton asked.

"Not bad for someone with two heart valves and rectal cancer."

My eyes opened wide.

Our being here at all was unlikely. I had been trying to eat healthy—organic vegetable soups, whole-wheat bread, salmon. For a change I had decided to indulge in a treat—a turkey burger with Duggan's famous sauce. At least that's why I thought we had come.

"Thirty-four years ago I was given six months to live," Larry said. In his twenties he was diagnosed with rectal cancer and had undergone fifty-five doses of cobalt radiation. "Radiation works," he said. Years later he fell off Duggan's roof and received several screws in his ankle and more stitches in his head. Later still he underwent heart surgery. Recently, his rectal cancer had returned. He was being treated again, was optimistic again.

Cancer patients relish survival stories. I learned to seek out positive examples and avoid the rest. For a few years, if someone famous contracted cancer and CNN ran a feature on it, I switched the channel. If a conversation seemed headed toward the grave, I put up my hand and said, as politely as I could, I only want to hear good cancer stories. The fear would diminish over time, but it slept lightly.

"You have no idea how grateful I am to hear that story," I said.

"My body looks like Frankenstein's. All that's missing are the screws in my jaw. But I'm still taking care of my family. And I'm still around."

He smacked the table with his fist. "My goal is to die being hit by a beer truck in our parking lot."

Up north again, we dined at the Grey Gables in Charlevoix with Andy, Amy and Alexis. My stomach felt queasy. I couldn't eat my maple-glazed salmon, a dish I usually loved.

"Hang in there," Burton said. "You'll be fine."

Andy said, "Mom isn't a child, Dad. You don't have to give her a pep talk."

"Dad's my coach," I said. "He's just doing his job."

When Andy played football during his senior year at Cranbrook, he was a center, co-captain of the team. I brought an absurdly-loud, old brass school bell to every home game. The bell had belonged to Burton's late mother, Edith. She rang it to summon her kids from the beach for lunch on summer days at their vacation house on Lake Erie near Rondeau Park, Ontario.

The clang resounded throughout the bleachers. I received glares from parents of the opposing football team whenever I rang the bell, which was any time our team did something remotely worthwhile.

Andy nodded. "I get it, Dad. Keep it up."

Later that night, queasiness turned into diarrhea and vomiting. Fear knifed through me. Stomach cancer, I thought. Once you're diagnosed with cancer, you lose the rational explanations that once comforted you. Minor symptoms seem deadly.

I hated to keep bothering Dr. Malone. Burton insisted.

"It's not cancer," Dr. Malone said. "It's probably the flu. Try Pepto Bismol or Imodium. You should feel better in the morning."

Thankfully, he was right once again. By morning my stomach had settled.

CHAPTER 8

Loving Eyes

We become habituated to reaching for something to ease the edginess of the moment. Thus we become less and less able to reside with even the most fleeting uneasiness or discomfort. … This is our way of trying to make life predictable.

—Pema Chodron, *Comfortable with Uncertainty*

AFTER MY FIRST chemotherapy treatment, Burton had said, "I don't think you should visit your mother while you're in chemo. That place is a breeding ground for germs." Whether or not he was right about the conditions in Mom's apartment building, he was in charge of my case. I'm ashamed to say I welcomed the excuse. I called Mom daily but for several weeks, stayed away.

Retired from fashion, my friend Brenda had trained with self-help guru Debbie Ford to be a relationship coach. Brenda theorized that part of my illness was caused by strained relations with my mother.

"I know she upsets you," Brenda said.

Mom refused to leave her apartment. Witnessing her self-imposed isolation depressed me.

"I hate how she refuses to have a life."

"We need to do a healing."

A bubble of dread worked its way from my stomach to my throat.

I uttered a dubious, "Okay."

Five years before, Brenda had hosted my fifty-fifth birthday luncheon. She designed a birthday cake reproducing my *Better Homes and Gardens* cover shot. During the five years I worked as a regional design editor for Meredith, I scored numerous covers of special-interest publications. They were always a thrill. But the biggest thrill was winning the cover of the flagship magazine. Even better, I had been invited to Des Moines for a meeting of what headquarters deemed their "most productive regional editors." A group of talented, competitive colleagues sat in a darkened auditorium as Jean Lemmon, editor of the magazine, showed slides from recent issues. Then she said, "This is our next cover. It's the way we want our future covers to look." On a screen maybe twenty feet tall, appeared a giant image of the shot I had styled—a blue-and-white bedroom of the Sitners', who lived next door to our former house up north. It was my first look at that cover, and for the next month I got chills every time I passed a magazine stand. Brenda knew what that cover meant to me. In short, she knew me well.

When you are sick, you consider all sorts of theories as to how you got that way. One theory is emotional stress. If Brenda was willing to help me struggle through the tension with my mother, it was worth a try.

I told Burton about Brenda's suggestion.

He rolled his eyes.

Burton, Brenda and I trudged through the front door and past the planters of fake green leaves at Mom's senior citizen residence. My sister and I had moved her here, despite her objections, because of her disability. Ten years before, she was chronologically young for such living quarters, though her physical needs demanded it. Now eighty-one, she was the age of many other occupants. In the lobby, a man played the piano. Several residents sat around singing "Yes, Sir, That's My Baby." Some lounged in wheelchairs; some had walkers beside them.

A man in a blue jogging suit with wispy, white hair pounded his cane in time to the music. Again I regretted that Mom, who enjoyed music and once loved being with people, refused to socialize.

In the elevator, I closed my eyes and took a deep breath, anticipating the stale odor ahead. Maybe because it was never unoccupied or aired out, Mom's apartment smelled to me like old athletic shoes. Walking down the hall to Mom's front door, I warned Brenda. "Take a breath."

Stepping into the foyer, I tried to breathe through my mouth. The odor still penetrated. "See what I mean?"

Brenda cocked her head. "I don't smell anything."

I raised my eyebrows and looked at Burton. "Neither do I," he said.

Mom's disability seemed to reawaken feelings of insecurity she had struggled with much of her life. She was born blind in one eye. As a young woman, she was fitted for a glass eye which made her appear normal. Looking a little like Jackie Kennedy, Mom was pretty but didn't think so. She grew up feeling unappreciated by her glamorous parents. My grandfather, a real-estate broker and developer, was tall with wavy, white hair. My grandmother had skin like the ripest peach. Her home was filled with antiques including a red lacquer chest that once belonged to the Duke of Marlborough. Mom, her sister and brother were mostly raised by governesses. Their parents spent several weeks a year on cruises to Europe, as many affluent Americans did in those days. Their frequent absences added to Mom's insecurity. She grew up determined to be attentive to her children and devoted herself to Anne and me. Raising two accomplished daughters helped improve her sense of worth. She called us the "lights" of her life.

Mom sat in her wheelchair at the end of the French Provincial-style wood dining table she'd had for decades. She wore one of several lightweight cotton, sleeveless plaid shirts I had bought her a few years before. She often felt hot. This was the one top she found comfortable. With my fashion background, I was convinced I could find other shirts she might enjoy. I kept shopping. She kept rejecting. Her artificial eye had become so uncomfortable that she no longer wore it. She kept that eyelid closed when people looked at her.

When Burton and I were working through our marriage crisis, we studied *A Course in Miracles* together. The course teaches that all human emotions can be reduced to two: love and fear. Fear, it contends, is an illusion. Love is all that's real.

Walking into Mom's apartment, I reminded myself to view my mother through loving eyes. I bent down to kiss her cool, dry cheek. She still had fine, high cheekbones.

Before Mom's disastrous foot surgery, there was a period when her self-confidence bloomed. By her mid-sixties, Mom was divorced from Dad and also from Larry, her second husband, a New Yorker. Larry proved attentive but broke, and had neglected to mention his chronic health problem and his lack of a real job. While she could still afford it, Mom divorced him and moved back to suburban Detroit from Manhattan. She was living on her own for the first time.

For several years during Mom's independent phase we had a tradition. On Mother's Day we visited the Greenfield Village Antiques Show in Dearborn, Michigan, and bought her a gift. We both loved antiques, though I preferred more primitive American pieces and Mom, more formal English ones. The annual show, held in Lovett Hall, included furniture and accessories sold by some of the country's top dealers. It raised funds for an indoor/outdoor museum complex featuring delights such as a Model T Ford, the Wright Brothers' bicycle shop and a working farm from the 1880s. Mom had once led my Brownie troop through the farm, and we'd watched candles and soap being made by ladies in long dresses, aprons and bonnets.

Mom's favorite dealer, Taylor Williams, specialized in the eighteenth-century English enameled boxes she adored. She referred to them as Battersea, named for a factory in Battersea, England, which produced them in the mid-1700s, though for several decades many other factories around Britain made them as well. My grandmother began collecting Battersea boxes many years before on her trips to Europe. Mom had inherited much of her mother's collection of enameled fruits and animals and snuff boxes painted with faux finishes, patterns, messages or pastoral scenes.

One Sunday we drove to Dearborn. I thought about how Mom seemed to have overcome much of the insecurity that had plagued her and how glad I was to witness it. I said, "You should be proud of yourself. You're living on your own in a beautiful apartment. You're hosting dinner parties. Dating a few men."

She said, "Imagine me—a geriatric Jezebel."

I laughed. Before her foot problem, Mom had a dazzling wit.

"You're playing bridge and golf. Working part time. Busy with friends. You're managing your investments."

"My best friends at the moment are Mr. Dow and Mr. Jones."

Mom invested conservatively, followed her stocks and spoke to her broker at least once a week. She had inherited real estate from her father. Some properties had been sold; others still brought in income. Mom rented a spacious two-bedroom apartment in Birmingham. Her designer-friend and bridge partner, Bill, helped her decorate. A French blue-and-white, abstract floral print covered a sofa and love seat. Mom adored blue and white. An old country French wood chest of drawers sat against one wall of the living room. On top, Mom displayed her collection of Battersea boxes, artfully arranged.

Mom was determined to pass on a financial inheritance to her daughters. That day in the car she said, "I want you and Anne to have something when I go to that Great Golf Course in the Sky. When I do, cremate me and scatter my ashes over Somerset Mall. Then I know you'll visit."

Somerset Mall was my favorite place to shop. Neiman Marcus occupied one end; Saks, the other. Neimans replaced earlier tenant, Bonwit Teller. Mom had once created events and handled publicity for Bonwits, her favorite of several part-time jobs.

Mom was in fine form that Mother's Day. She was working for the Feigenson/ Preston Gallery, representing emerging artists, many from Detroit, and owned by my friend Mary Preston. Mom didn't make much money, but she enjoyed feeling that she was helping artists. She loved her apartment and her little indoor garden in front of a large window, with a Ficus tree and pots of flowering begonias, one resting on an antique brass stand. She was in her sixties. She hadn't yet been diagnosed with Parkinson's or undergone the foot surgery that would end her ability to ever stroll around an antiques show again.

As we got out of the car, I felt that little swoosh of anticipation I always felt when entering an antiques show. I slowed my pace to match Mom's. She wore shoes with crepe wedge soles. In future years I wondered if her preference for this type of shoe shortened her calf muscles and contributed to the problem she had with her toe surgery. I would never know. Mom and I headed to Taylor's booth. The air smelled of cloves and dried orange peel. The murmur of happy conversation rose from the booths we passed. Overhead lights brought forth a sheen from china plates and vases, brass candlesticks and polished furniture.

Taylor stood behind a glass case, looking elegant in a grey cashmere sweater. Inside the case, dozens of small, colorful enamel-on-copper boxes nested like jewels. He looked up we approached.

"Barbara," Taylor exclaimed, smiling broadly, taking her hand. "How is my favorite collector?"

"Fine," Mom said. "And how is my favorite dispenser of vintage baloney?"

"Superb, now that I see you." He raised his eyebrows and lowered his voice. "I have new temptations."

"Be still, my fluttering heart."

Taylor took out a delicate little round pink object. "A patch box," he said. "Patches were beauty spots, popular in Georgian times." We always learned from Taylor. Mom nodded. I could tell this wasn't the one. He took out an oval tube. "An etui, or needle case," he said. "Needles were called bodkins."

Mom looked at several other boxes, then pointed to one shaped like a walnut. Taylor showed it to her. It was light brown with darker brown lines where the crevices of a real walnut would be. "I'm nuts about it," she said. "How much? For your favorite collector?"

"I need to check my inventory. See what I paid. How much room I have."

This stall tactic was part of the mating ritual. It gave the collector time to fall in love and to reassure herself of the dealer's integrity. Taylor checked some numbers hand-written into a ledger.

"Hmm," he said. "From a fine estate in the Berkshires."

Sandhill cranes, which Burton and I see in Florida and in northern Michigan, have a dramatic mating ritual. These gawky, grey birds, up to five feet tall, squawk together in a vocalization known as unison calling, a gobble primordial enough to conjure visions of 100 million years ago when dinosaurs roamed the earth. To attract each other, sandhill cranes throw back their heads and sing and dance and flap their wings and leap up and down. The mating ritual at an antiques show is more subtle. In a confidential voice, the dealer mentions the recent source of a piece. Citing provenance is part of the foreplay. It adds romance, prepares the collector for consummation at a higher price.

"It's in perfect condition," Taylor said. He opened and closed the lid. "It's marked $625. I can do a little better. $575."

"For a thief, you're a charmer," Mom said. She asked him to hold the box for her. "I want to discuss matters with my investment adviser." She nodded at me then patted her stomach. "This old bodkin needs sustenance."

We headed for the lunchroom, smelled the aroma of warm pie crust, and decided on chicken pot pies.

"The box is charming," I said. "You don't have anything like it. Offer $500. He'll come back at $550. Compromise at $525. I'll split it with you." Bargaining was part of the process. Even at the best of shows.

A few years later, recovering from her broken leg, Mom stayed in what was considered the best convalescent home in the city. Anything she wasn't wearing was stolen. We didn't want the same fate to befall Mom's beloved Battersea boxes. When we moved her to The Trowbridge, with Mom's permission, Anne and I divided up the collection. The exchange was bittersweet. Anne and I were glad to have the boxes but sad that Mom could no longer enjoy them every day. I had a glass-front display case built for my half of the collection, including the $525 walnut. The case hangs on the powder room wall of our Franklin house.

The night of Brenda's attempted healing, I glanced around at traces of my mother's former life. In the living/dining room, there was a small print by Miró with a splotch of purple and a little Milton Avery etching of the beach—Mom loved the ocean. A Frankenthaler print washed with tan and teal-blue hung above the dining table. Mom enjoyed modern art and once worked as an assistant in Detroit's renowned Gertrude Kasle Gallery. I inherited my love of art from my mother.

I tried to ignore the dust on the chrome-and-glass cocktail table, the chips in the blue-and-white Dr. Wall porcelain ashtrays, the black wheelchair marks on the walls, the frayed arms of the blue-and-white sofa and loveseat. The fabric had been discontinued. I had brought over many samples of new blue-and-white fabrics to reupholster the seating. Mom didn't like any of them. An overgrown Ficus tree dropped leaves in the corner near the balcony.

Burton slumped in a light-blue, antique wing chair in the far corner of the living room. Brenda asked me to sit at the dining table with my mother and to hold her hand. I had inherited my mother's small, delicate hands.

Brenda told my mother about the training she had received. She said, "Barbara, talk about your relationship with Suzy."

Mom hesitated. Seconds seemed to stretch apart, like bubblegum under your shoe. I looked at my mother's hand. I always wore a sheer, neutral nail polish which I applied myself—practical because it lasted a week and didn't show chips. Mom used to wear a pale, pinkish-apricot shade. Now her fingernails were bare; her hands, bumpy and bent from arthritis.

Mom spoke slowly, as though under water. I don't know if her halting speech was caused by her Parkinson's or her many medications. Or by what she had to say.

"I don't think Suzy loves me."

"Tell Suzy," Brenda said.

She looked at me. "I don't think you love me."

Compassion, I reminded myself. Loving eyes. Still I tasted resentment on the back of my tongue. A taste all the more bitter because now I knew how it felt to be sick and vulnerable, and still I felt angry. Angry at Mom for withdrawing from life. My witty, outgoing mother had been replaced by a fearful, stubborn recluse. And knowing how devoted Mom had been to her daughters, I felt all the more guilty and ashamed for not being more understanding.

It wasn't so much the deterioration of Mom's body that depressed me. I would go for a walk or to a restaurant and see people in wheelchairs, getting out and carrying on with their lives. What troubled me was how Mom had given up. In recent years, she had even refused to come to our house for Thanksgiving dinner with the family, although David and Andy would drive her and help her in and out of the car. Her self-imposed incarceration had gone on for more than ten years. I once heard a psychologist mention something he called "compassion fatigue." I realized, with dismay, he described what was happening to me.

"You felt the same way about your mother and your father and your husband," I said. "You can't feel loved if you don't love yourself."

Mom gave me a sad, frozen stare. She seemed to want to say more but couldn't find the words.

"Suzy," Brenda said, "What do you need to tell your mother?"

"Anne and I couldn't leave you where you were. You were too isolated. We found and fixed up the nicest place we could for you. We hoped you would adjust to being here. You won't even try."

Mom continued to stare at me. I wiped my cheeks.

"I feel like I've let you down," I said. "I've always wanted to make you proud."

Slowly, Mom said, "I'm proud of both my girls."

Brenda asked, "Barbara, what do you need from Suzy?"

She hesitated and seemed to frown, though her face no longer showed much expression. I still feel sorrow when I think about her simple request.

"Just to tell me she loves me."

Mom used to write poems for peoples' birthdays. Living in downtown Birmingham, she wrote a limerick about endless road construction on Woodward Avenue. The poem, so clever that I saved it, was published in *The Eccentric*, the local newspaper. It ended with Mom's typical humor:

> No more Band-Aids for Woodward.
> This is the real thing, albeit.
> They say they'll finish in the fall.
> I hope I live to see it!

When I was a girl, Mom drove me to ice-skating lessons and art classes. She conducted family "mystery trips" to the circus and the zoo. When I turned forty, Mom threw me a birthday luncheon. Foam core typewriter centerpieces had daisies popping out where the piece of paper would be. Guests wore buttons that read: Suzy's Our Type.

Mom wore her Santa Claus hat with the jingle bell to the Christmas dinners she hosted at her apartment. She prepared rare roast beef, Anne's and my favorite, and arranged shiny, red-and-silver Christmas ornaments in a blue-and-white bowl in the center of the table. The table where she now sat, shrunken, in her wheelchair. Her left foot flopped to the side despite the bulky, navy-blue boot meant to straighten it. A full-time aide waited in the next room.

I pushed the words out. "I love you, Mom."

"Suzy," Brenda said, "What do you need from your mother?"

"I need to focus on getting well. I need to let go of my sense of responsibility for you, Mom. I need you to be okay with that."

"I'm okay," Mom said.

Home later, I thought about what Mom had said. I loved her and always would. But it was hard to accept that this withdrawn, diminished stranger was my mother. I wished she could have been her old, lively self again. I wished I could have been more gracious and tolerant.

Our kids joined us for dinner that night. I was grateful for their energy, grateful to again see how vital and engaged they were. We sat in a circle, held hands and recited the Jewish prayer for healing.

Parkinson's, and the medicines for it, can take over a person's body and spirit. I still don't know if my mother's fearfulness resulted from early-childhood wounding, from an acquired lack of confidence, from disease or drugs or disability, or from anger over the move we forced her to make. I do know I desperately hoped to never be a mother my kids would have to worry about. Mom was dealt a tough hand. Earlier in her life, she may have felt the same way.

So many matters are beyond our control. I had inherited several of my mother's traits. Her sense of humor. Her curiosity. Her appreciation for travel, for books and for language. I prayed I would never fall into as dark and lonely a place as Mom had, that I would never become so defeated. Feeling needy, I realized, was one of the toughest parts of my illness.

I remained unsettled about the visit. We did not reach the breakthrough Brenda hoped for. I didn't feel healed, and I'm sure Mom didn't either. We both stayed stuck in our stances of resentment. Silence is self-perpetuating. Resentment is more than a splinter, easily removed with needle and tweezers and a deft hand. Resentment lodges deep, in a pit that is hard to reach.

Mom would continue to decline. We wouldn't have the time or place or heart for further healing sessions. Less than two years later, Mom died at eighty-three. Admiring her Battersea collection takes me back to our Mother's Day outings. It helps me remember the mom I want to remember, the mom she'd want me to remember.

In the years since, I have come to see that Mom and I did the best we could in all the stages of our relationship, the happier stretches and those that were more problematic. I've become more forgiving of both of us. No one could have predicted the complication that occurred with Mom's toe surgery. When Anne and I moved her apartment, she gave up. I'm sure she berated herself every day for the medical choice she made. I have asked myself hundreds of times, if Anne and I could change our decision to move Mom's residence, would we? Considering all the factors, I still cannot come up with a better solution.

As for Brenda's attempted healing that night, at least I know we tried.

Almost two months into my cancer fight, I had been spending a lot of time talking to God, but wasn't yet aware of the ways in which God talked to me. Marianne, I would come to see, was one of those ways. She called. I told her what I was going through—surgery, chemo and radiation, all within six weeks.

"I feel guilty feeling sorry for myself when I've been so blessed up to now and when others have worse problems. And I'm afraid if I don't think positively, I'll get even sicker."

Marianne sighed. "You sound mad at yourself for being sick. You need to be more loving."

At that time, Marianne Williamson was serving as a minister for the Unity church in the Detroit area. We had become friends. Her sermons and best-selling books had comforted me before. She had introduced Burton and me to *A Course in Miracles*, which opened a path to revive our marriage. She had written the foreword to *Back from Betrayal*. Now she helped me see how hard I was being on myself.

"This illness is an emotional catastrophe," she said. "There's no need to pretend otherwise. Don't mask this horror in the name of positive thinking. This is a chance to release decades of fear-based thinking. Suppressing fear doesn't get rid of it. Let the fear out."

Counseling AIDS patients, Marianne had come up with an exercise. She advised patients to write letters to their disease and to allow a response from the viewpoint of their disease.

"They learned some interesting things," she said. "You might find it helpful."

"Maybe," I said. At the moment, I was too physically and emotionally drained. And too afraid to confront my disease head on.

Marianne's suggestion stayed with me for the rest of the day. That evening, though still doubtful, I picked up my pen. By the time I put my journal down, I was trembling. My disease seemed smarter than I was.

> *Cancer:*
> *I hate what you've done to me. I hate how you have invaded my body and taken control of my activities and my energy. I hate the strain you've put on my relationship with Burton, my inability to travel, to laugh, to do things for others. I hate being so absorbed in myself. I hate how you've robbed me of trust in my body. I hate how silently and malevolently you snuck up on me and changed everything. I hate you, cancer!*
> *… Thanks for nothing. I want you out of my body, out of my head, out of my life. I want my life, my body, my health back.*
> *Suzy*

The response:

> *Dear Suzy,*
> *I'm not trying to punish you—only to exist. I know you are fighting me on every front. You have faith*

in your doctors and are trying to believe in your-
self, to muster your own courage and endurance, to
believe that God will see you through.

I know some other things. You worry too much and
need to let God take over. You need to trust that
everything happens for a reason, whether or not
you understand.

If you beat me in this battle, I'll have a chance to
teach you important lessons:

To stop being such a worrier.

To stay in the present.

To better appreciate the abundance in your life.

For your sake, I hope I'm a temporary inconve-
nience. I hope you'll someday look back after I'm
gone and say, "Thanks, cancer, for teaching me to
live more fully and for bringing me more awareness
of my soul's purpose."

Until then, you'll have to live with uncertainty and
with your inability to control circumstances (an
illusion in the first place). You'll have to live, too,
with the blow to your ego and your image, with the
fact that you're as vulnerable as anyone else and
not as tough or independent as you thought.

You and Burton came through one excruciating
problem with grace. You'll just have to try again,
with his patient and loving support, to come
through another.

I am not your fault. I just am.

I know you've lost dear friends to cancer and have
seen how it ate away their bodies. I know this pros-
pect scares you. For your sake, I hope you won't
join them. You're in for some rough months. Hope-
fully, you'll defeat me and go on to lead a life that
is healthier from all I've taught you. I am a tough
teacher.

Keep fighting. Show me what you've got.
Cancer

When we built our house in Franklin eight years before, I named it Acorn Hill in honor of the many acorns scattered on our ridge. I loved the idea of acorns and their big-league prospects. I designed ceramic acorn tiles to be set into the cherry wood panel above the library fireplace and bronze acorn pulls with little ridged caps for cabinet doors. I delighted in small touches. I had written about other peoples' beautiful homes for years. This was the first residence I'd lived in that expressed my creativity.

On one wall of the library, cherry wood bookshelves extended to the ceiling and spanned the doorway. They contained books on art and travel and my grandmother's out-of-print books on antique porcelains. They displayed a small, ceramic Picasso plate depicting a mask, a multiple we'd bought on a trip to the south of France. There was a primitive wood carving of the fighter Joe Louis, one of Burton's heroes. I had spotted the figure at a folk-art show in New York and brought him back to the state where he grew up. There were books on Albert Kahn.

Kahn, my late great-uncle, was the architect whose modern designs enabled Henry Ford to develop the assembly line. He created hundreds of factories in Michigan and around the world, including in Russia. Many of those factories were converted to build tanks during World War II, helping to defeat the Nazis. Kahn also designed beautiful homes and office buildings in the Detroit area. Among them, the Fisher Building (named for the original Fisher Brothers who started General Motors), now run by our sons. I was proud to be named for Albert's sister, my grandmother Mollie. Mollie is my middle name. I like to think a love for design is in my DNA.

In our library, I had written holiday letters and thank you notes and addressed invitations. Here we had shared drinks with friends and viewed the videotape of Andy's wedding. Now Burton slumped into a cinnabar chenille sofa, feet on the beige, travertine marble-topped coffee table, worn-out size 13 Rockport loafers on the floor beside him. The TV chattered in the background.

I sat on the floor beside my husband, next to the coffee table. We had bought it for the family room of our first house, a small colonial in Huntington Woods. I remember the circumstances of buying furniture the way others remember where they were when Kennedy was shot. We moved to "the Woods" from Detroit in 1971, the year David was born, four years after the Detroit riots. I was pregnant; we wanted a safe neighborhood in which to walk our baby—a response characteristic of the "white flight" that occurred after the uprisings. The riots took place in 1967, the year we got married. We witnessed them in person. With my typical desire to be part of the action, I insisted we drive to 12th Street and Grand River Avenue to see what was happening. With shock and dismay, we watched mobs of people hurling bricks through store windows and dashing off with merchandise and upending parked cars as though participants in some macabre sporting event. I wrote a front-page story about the retail impact of the riots for *Home Furnishings Daily*. My research led me to a man whose carpet warehouse had burned down and for whom Burton found new space. Burton had begun to bring in more real-estate commissions for Schostak Bros. He would go on to manage the brokerage division. David was born soon after we moved. Later, I took a consulting job for an ad agency representing Gantos, a chain of Michigan fashion stores, since closed. My earnings at the time paid for the caramel leather Eames chair which now sat across from me and for the travertine marble-topped coffee table on which I spread photos of family and friends.

I sorted the last six months worth of pictures into piles, from the oldest to the latest. Since early in our marriage, I had filled nearly two dozen black, pigskin, loose-leaf binder albums. I designed library shelves deep enough for the albums, which bore dates on their spines and now took up two shelves. I updated them every six months and felt satisfied when I finished adding the most recent photos. If I wanted to remember when we traveled to Hong Kong or Buenos Aires or who had attended a party, I leafed through my albums. In recent years, many people stored photos online, in some vast, intangible e-space. Even if I were talented with a computer, which I'm not, I still preferred my albums. Outdated as they had become, I liked their heft and presence. They were a memory of good times and good people and a visible record of our history. A sign that we loved and lived. That we celebrated. That we mattered. As weak and worried as I currently felt, I was all the more determined to keep them up.

I studied a photo from the surprise party I gave for Burton a few months before. I never wanted a surprise party. I liked to look forward to special events. But over the years, when we were invited to other peoples' surprise parties, Burton had insisted he liked the idea. In February, I had thrown a surprise party for his sixty-first birthday at Morel's restaurant in Southfield. I had searched the Internet for cowboy-themed decorations and impressed myself by finding boot-shaped candles and cardboard, barroom swinging doors. Burton remained unaware until we walked through the dimly-lit restaurant and he spotted the barroom doors in back, mounted at the party-room entrance. "What have you done?" he said.

The party room was a happy jumble of cowboy hats, red bandanas, straw, sunflowers and white helium balloons printed with cow-like black spots. About sixty close friends and family in western boots and suede vests and denim jeans and skirts offered hugs and greetings. Many gave toasts. There were golf stories. Horse stories. Dad stories. Andy talked about consulting with Burton every morning and about how glad he was that Burton didn't object when he ignored his advice. David talked about Burton's passion for horses and cowboy movies and John Wayne. And about how his father knew almost every word from *Lonesome Dove*. He said, "Up north, with favorite guests, my dad quotes *The Man from Snowy River*: 'You're welcome at my campfire any time.' Dad, get a new line!" Mike Duggan, an executive with Wayne County, talked about his pride in the county headquarters building that Burton had redeveloped and restored. Burton's old friend Michael, who introduced us, recalled an incident from their young teens. Burton bet him he could not move his aunt's car one inch. Michael turned the key, accelerated, and crashed into the garage wall.

In the photo I held, Burton wore one of his favorite beige, felt cowboy hats which we'd secretly brought along for him. He looked so happy. I felt grateful I had thrown the party while I had a chance. Otherwise, on my deathbed, which loomed larger than it once had, I might have regretted that some future spouse would throw my husband's surprise party. I pasted the photo down and squeezed four more party photos onto the same page.

I pasted down a photo of my sister, my book publicist, Grace, and me at my book-launch press luncheon at La Côte Basque in New York. My peppy smile covered up plenty of anxiety. I worried that telling our story could harm our business and our reputation, which our sons were working so hard to build. That it would damage my mother's already-fragile feelings and cause strain with my husband and children. Those worries, so pressing at the time, had been upstaged by my cancer diagnosis.

I turned to Burton. "I've been thinking," I said.

In the past, if he were reading a paper or watching a movie on TV, my husband would try to ignore me. He might mutter, "Wait 'til I'm done with this article" or "Wait 'til this part is over." Now he put down the paper, lowered the TV volume, and gazed at me.

"It's always been my job to ask the medical questions and read the books and figure out the best doctors," I said. "I feel like I've let you down. I'm sorry for putting so much pressure on you."

He shook his head. "Don't apologize on my account," he said. "Over the years, there were nights I'd lie awake, tossing and sweating and worrying about business. You stayed up with me, helping me to talk things through. You always kept your head. Your belief gave me confidence I could work things out."

The real-estate business was full of risks, competition and legal and financial subtleties. Market and tax considerations kept changing. I didn't know how to advise my husband. The best I could do was to reassure him. We had taken the same approach with our children. When they faced decisions, we supported their ability to choose. Though some friends considered us too liberal, we believed if our sons made their own choices, they'd be more invested in making them work. They learned from their mistakes. They each determined the camps and schools they attended. Andy opted for private school; David, public. I think they made the right choices. They did so more often than not.

There was an added dimension to the confidence I appeared to display in a crisis. I was afraid of too much emotion. Because I saw my mother take things so personally, I veered the other way. I dodged painful feelings. Some people drink or take drugs to escape from worry. Staying busy was how I avoided bigger, scarier forces. The list of possibilities for doom was endless. My children occupied at least the top ten spots. Would they remain healthy? Sober? Out of trouble? Would they stay awake at the wheel? I had friends who had lost children. We were no more immune than they were to such an incomprehensible loss. Could a bad real-estate deal bankrupt us? Would my husband stay faithful? What if our house caught fire? If the stock market crashed? If a terrorist got his hands on a nuclear bomb? And, oh by the way, cancer. When I was involved in a project—creating a centerpiece, writing an article, working a crossword puzzle, reading a book, updating an album—my brain didn't have time to wallow in the what-ifs. Now I wondered if my calm façade covered up such a cesspool of worries that I'd made myself sick. In spite of my busyness, I'd been walloped with a monster what-if.

"This is the first time I've seen you so tuned-in," Burton said. "I'm not scared of your feelings. This experience is an emotional drain on both of us. But it's not an inconvenience. We're both getting used to a new normal. We'll never have carefree years again. But our new normal is powerful. We'll enjoy experiences differently than before."

"I wonder if I ever had carefree days," I said.

"You've drunk from a lot of half-empty glasses. Maybe this experience will help you see differently."

"I hope so," I said, and could not stop myself from adding, "I should live so long."

I was economical in the photos I displayed. And choosy. Subjects had to look good. I only showcased the best. Keeping up appearances mattered. How I wrote and published a memoir in which neither my husband nor I looked very good still baffled me.

Normally I bought two photo albums at a time. I could fit up to two years' worth of photos in each book. The last time I went to buy albums at Green's Art Supply in Birmingham, the salesperson told me the books were being discontinued. In an uncharacteristic show of extravagance, I purchased eighteen, plus several packages of refills.

I pasted down a picture of me in a yellow leather jacket, standing at a podium, reading from *Back from Betrayal* at Border's in Birmingham. Now I had a yet another new worry. I hoped I hadn't wasted my money. I wondered how many more albums I'd get to fill.

CHAPTER 9

Whatever Arises

This is another day, O Lord. I know not what
it will bring forth, but make me
ready, Lord, for whatever it may be.

—**Book of Common Prayer**

"**I'M GOING TO** enjoy every damn day," Arnie said.

Our mutual friend Barbara insisted I call. Barbara and Arnie volunteered at a cancer center in Miami. Arnie had recovered from endometrial stromal sarcoma, cancer of the connective tissue, different from my type of uterine cancer, but equally rare. Following a hysterectomy and radiation, Arnie was given a fifty-fifty chance of survival. After two years without a recurrence, her chances had risen to seventy-five percent.

"I believe a positive attitude helps my immune system. I see myself surrounded with white light. I refuse to throw out a good day just because I had some bad ones," she said.

I hung up with Arnie feeling impressed by her courage. She reeled off her survival numbers like someone rattling off the pounds she'd lost at a Weight Watchers meeting. She said that during treatment she came home and napped for hours. If I could sleep, I thought, I might feel more positive, too. I had slept poorly since my twenties. The problem worsened when my oncologist took me off hormones.

Seeking slumber, in past years I tried countless approaches. I downed melatonin and tryptophan supplements. I kept sleep journals, charted whether coffee or alcohol or chocolate made a difference. I tried reading in bed and not reading in bed. Going to bed later or earlier. Maintaining a regular bedtime. Cooling the room. TV on. TV off. Exercise. Prayer. Meditation. Hot baths. Tylenol PM. Antihistamines. Xanax. Welbutrin. Ativan. Zoloft. Nothing worked. My brain refused to settle down. Ambien helped me fall asleep but not stay asleep. Sonata and Lunesta produced the same short-term result, despite the model with perfect hair snoozing on TV. I read books and articles on sleep, discussed my problem with a leading authority. Still, I felt wired. Most nights I tossed and turned. Now, in those rare moments when I did doze off, I awoke from a sleeping nightmare to a living one.

Listening to the radio, I heard a doctor say something chilling: Our bodies release healing hormones when we sleep. I had struggled through a logic course in college. I didn't get much farther than comprehending what happens when A equals B. A: If I wasn't sleeping, then B: I wasn't helping my body to heal. I grew more desperate to find a solution.

Before cancer, I had never taken antidepressants. During the lowest moments of our marriage problems, I resisted. I hated the thought of depending on pills. But cancer attacks your spirit as well as your body. I was willing to try anything to help me smile again.

A friend told me about an antidepressant drug that enhanced serotonin release. I met with a psychopharmacologist. Dr. Waldman said the drug had been on the market for several years. If it worked, she said, it would help me sleep at night, give me energy in the daytime, and improve my mood.

"What's the downside?"

"Patients complain it increases their appetite. They go off it when they put on too much weight. But you lost several pounds during surgery. You could stand to gain a few."

I doubted this new drug would work any better than the many other remedies I had tried. But that night I swallowed a round tablet, the size of a capital O, the color of Dijon mustard. I also took 5mg of Ambien. When I awoke the next morning, a miracle had occurred. The clock read 6 a.m.

My appetite did increase. Within several weeks, I regained the few pounds I had lost from my hysterectomy and had to refrain from eating everything I wanted. I considered the self-denial a fair price for the gift of sleep and the brighter outlook that comes with it.

I continue to take my chemical cocktail. I am not proud of being hooked on prescription drugs. Still, I am grateful to sleep eight hours most nights. Most days I speed walk or ride a bike to counteract my ambitious appetite. I hope my liver will forgive the added chemical burden. If my regimen stops working, I find comfort in the strides scientists are making in understanding brain chemistry. God willing, modern science will continue to help.

"The hardest part is not knowing," I said. "If I'll be around for Alexis' first day of school. If I'll get to hold all my grandchildren. If Burton will marry someone else."

Two months into my cancer struggle, the early-fall breeze and the western sun lighting up the porch could not settle my jagged nerves. I sat lamenting to Donna, a friend who had recently trained to become a psychologist and meditation teacher. I hadn't seen Donna in several years. Hearing I was sick, she just showed up one day. I still hadn't perceived how extraordinary it was that this kept happening, how when I was most vulnerable, the words or guidance I needed somehow kept appearing, as if by magic.

Donna told me about Indian Prince Siddhārtha Gautama who sat in a walled courtyard under a Bodhi tree 2,500 years ago. "He realized something so profound that he left the security of his parents' palace, took a vow of poverty, and became The Buddha."

"What did he realize?"

"Whatever arises is subject to cessation."

Cancer had thrown my life into chaos. I felt confused about the diagnosis, concerned about the treatment, anxious about the future, and unable to escape my negative thinking.

"How do I make fears subside?"

"Being swept away by emotion is a habit," Donna said in a voice as soothing as the swish of Lake Michigan on a summer day. "In meditation, we replace one habit with another: the ability to observe our thoughts. Visualize yourself as a surfer; your thoughts are waves. Detach from the thinking process. Don't connect to your thoughts, ride them."

Donna displayed a serenity I had seen once before. Thirty-some years earlier, as a reporter for the *Detroit News*, I interviewed Swami Satchidananda, the founder of Integral Yoga. Our encounter didn't take place at an ashram in far-off India but rather in a meeting room of the Book Cadillac Hotel in downtown Detroit. It wasn't the Swami's long, white beard or soft gaze that drew me—it was his aura. As a journalist, I interviewed hundreds of people and forgot many of them. I never forgot the radiance that surrounded the Swami.

"All thoughts are equal," Donna said. "Through meditation, we practice mindful awareness. We give our thoughts the tender, non-judgmental label: thinking. We detach from them and let them go. When we meditate long enough, we become so familiar with our thoughts that we learn to befriend them. We say hello anger, or jealousy or fear. And we say goodbye."

Donna recommended I read Pema Chodron, an American Buddhist nun. The next afternoon, I found *Comfortable with Uncertainty*, a jewel of a book, nested in a gift bag on my front porch. The book teaches mind training (*Lojong* in Tibetan) and the practice of taking and sending (*tonglen* in Tibetan), that is, taking *in* pain and sending *out* pleasure. Pema's essays were brilliant in their simplicity. Occasionally they were even comforting.

I am an avid reader. An author becomes my friend. Snuggling in bed with a book is like having the author all to myself on her smartest, most insightful day. Pema Chodron remains on the shelf right beside my bed.

My physical reactions worsened. At 11 p.m., I could not stop shaking. My heart pounded like a jackhammer breaking cement. Burton pressed a thermometer into my mouth. He checked the clock. Three minutes later he put on reading glasses.

"101. Call Dr. Malone."

Karmanos doctors encourage patients to call at any hour. When I experienced unfamiliar, frightening sensations, it helped to know my doctor would speak to me within minutes.

"This doesn't sound like a reaction to chemo or radiation," Dr. Malone said. "You could be hypoglycemic. Tell Burt to make you a milkshake."

Burton raced to the kitchen. I heard the banging of doors and the whirr of a blender. I heard footsteps speeding back. Burton thrust out a glass of foamy, white liquid smelling of vanilla.

"Drink," he said.

A thick, cold sweetness coated my tongue. I kept swallowing. Within seconds, my trembling stopped; my temperature dropped. Terror subsided into low-grade concern. Once again, I marveled at Dr. Malone's ability to diagnose what was wrong, even over the telephone. I hadn't even told him I had stopped eating sugar.

More strange symptoms followed. A few hours after my second chemo, my face turned red and itchy. I rubbed on cortisone cream. That night, I again felt miserable and frightened. My cheeks continued to itch. My body resumed shaking. I wrapped a blanket around me. Burton stuck a thermometer in my mouth. Back up to 101 degrees.

"Call," Burton said.

"Me again," I said.

"You're coming off steroids," Dr. Malone said. Steroids are given intravenously before chemo to prevent inflammation.

"Take Benadryl. Eat. Drink plenty of fluids. You should be better by tomorrow."

I was taking antibiotics for a bladder infection. Dr. Forman called to report on my urine culture.

"Abnormal," he said. "E. coli. Stay on Cipro."

Burton had planned to spend the next day up north. I wanted him to go. We had not been apart since I was diagnosed. Benadryl helped to lower my fever. But as I sat in bed that night, my heart continued to race.

"Maybe you shouldn't go," I said.

"What's wrong?"

"I don't think I'm going to make it."

"I'm calling Jon," Burton said.

"It's too late to call."

"I'm calling."

Jon, the donor of Chemo Bear, was one of Andy's best friends. He had undergone massive chemotherapy for testicular cancer a couple of years before. He not only survived, but fared so well that he'd moved to Chicago and begun Imerman's Angels, a cancer survivor-to-patient support group. Burton had compiled names to call in an emergency. Jon's topped his list.

"Some days were so bad I wanted to die," Jon said. "It took all I had just to make a lap around the island in our kitchen."

I told Jon about my ghosts. About Mickey, a sweet and beautiful friend, who had wasted away from lung cancer. About Marilyn, a vibrant neighbor who became a haggard skeleton before dying of melanoma. About Jackie, a gutsy art dealer, ravaged by breast cancer.

"All cancer patients have ghosts," Jon said. "Remembering them is part of the process. Your reactions are normal. The sun will shine again ... eventually."

It was after midnight when I calmed down enough to let Jon go to bed.

I took two Benadryls and dreamt about a wild rodent chasing Burton and me. I awoke, terrified and shaking. My eyes burned; my mouth felt dry. The rodent was chemotherapy, I thought. I was so frightened I didn't think I could survive any more chemo.

Stay in the moment, I told myself. I surveyed my body. Nothing really hurt.

I visited my grandmother in the hospital almost thirty years ago. She was in her eighties, dying of ovarian cancer, and overcome by depression. I remember saying, "We're all going to die someday." I wish I could take those words back.

The tree outside our bedroom is growing too close to the window and I don't have the strength to call anyone to trim it. I look in our calendar at dates we were supposed to have and feel so detached from things that once mattered.

Bobbye thought losing her hair was the worst part of cancer. I think it's the scariness of my body's reactions and the not-knowing. I feel like my faith is being tested, and I'm not measuring up. I am consumed by fear.

Burton lay in bed with me this morning and held me. It made me sad that instead of enjoying his loving attention, I could only think about losing it. I want my life back.

Someone named Donna Roberts said something that described my relationship with Brenda. "A friend is someone who, when you've forgotten the song in your heart, reminds you of the words." When you are ambushed by a cancer diagnosis, you wonder if you'll ever sing again. Brenda refused to let me forget the words.

Soon after my second chemo treatment, dozens of limp, brown strands began clinging to my pillow, and I didn't have many to begin with. Shiny, pink scalp began showing. Days before, Brenda had driven across town to share in a chemo rite of passage, a visit to a wig store. She'd supervised the photographing of my then-hairstyle, consulted on the cut of my future wig and chosen each blonde and brown shade that would comprise it.

Now Brenda drove me to our second visit. I was encouraged to see a beautiful redhead walk into the lobby carrying two wigs and apparently wearing a third. She was a former model. I had met her many years ago when I was a fashion editor. Her chin length bob had always looked perfect. It had never occurred to me that her hair wasn't technically her own. The wig shop we had chosen was reportedly the best in town. Seeing this model here confirmed it.

In a private room, I was seated in a beauty-salon chair. A young man got right to the business of shaving the hair that had stuck by me. Brenda held my hand. "I can't look," I whispered and squeezed my eyes shut. I smelled a floral scent of hairspray, felt a tickle on my skull, and heard the buzz of an electric razor. When the buzzing stopped, I peeked at the floor. A shaft of light fell on the dusting of brown and blonde hair that surrounded my chair. I raised my eyes, peered at my cold, pale, naked skull in the mirror, and sighed. I resembled someone from a concentration camp. I looked at Brenda. Her cheeks glistened.

The stylist lifted my new wig off a plastic form, shook it, pulled it over my head and jiggled it into place.

"Voilà," he said, clapping his hands. He stood back, appraising. "You have a great occipital bone."

Occipital bones aren't a feature like breasts that everyone appreciates. There are no C or D measurements to quantify occipital-bone protrusions. Designers create tank tops to show off cleavage. No one tailors hats to display occipital contours. Oprah doesn't do shows on fitting them. I never thought to admire my occipital bone. I had spent so much time lamenting my fine, thin hair, and suddenly I learned the real attraction lay underneath.

Brenda fingered my new wig with a professional air. She nodded and smiled at me. "Better than your own color."

The brown strands were real; the highlights, synthetic, the stylist said. "The blonde stays brighter that way." The wig would be trimmed and thinned to match my former hairstyle.

"Make it thicker," I said. "I might as well get something good out of this."

Soon after, Brenda returned with me for the final fitting. Regarding my wig perched on a white Styrofoam form, she said, "It looks like a Gertrude."

"Gertrude it is," I said.

I pulled the wig on. Brenda fluffed it with her hands and stood back, bending her head side to side, checking out my coiffure. She asked the stylist to taper it around the neck. He disappeared with it and returned in a few minutes to put the wig on my head again. The hair in back appeared to have been styled with a curling iron. It curved in nicely.

"It feels tight," I said.

"You'll get used to it," the stylist said.

I wore Gertrude home, admiring her several times in the car mirror. As pretty as she looked, she did continue to pinch.

Brenda advised me to have a second wig made for times when Gertrude was in service. Gertrude needed to be returned to the wig shop to be cleaned and styled.

"I'm not vain enough or extravagant enough," I said. My wig had cost more than $1,000. "I'll wear a scarf if I have to."

Most women, I have noticed, are dissatisfied with their hair. It is too curly or too straight, too thick or too thin, too grey, too wiry, too blah. I promise you this. Even if your hair frustrates or disappoints you; even if you slather it with volumizers and gels and plump it with Velcro rollers and hot-air blowers; even if you buoy it up with texturizers, all of which I have tried; even if stylists never attain the color you crave no matter how many magazine ads and celebrity photos you show them; even if you've never liked what passed for your hair before, you miss it when it's gone.

Though I brought her back several times to be adjusted, Gertrude remained slightly uncomfortable. I never did get used to the tightness. But on her good days, when she was freshly done, she was prettier than my own hair ever was, even at its very best when I had it done for my sons' weddings. Gertrude looked like the hair I envied in Clairol shampoo ads.

For most of the last forty years, every six weeks I had visited a salon in hopes of thickening and brightening my crowning glory, which mostly resulted in my crowning defeat. I thumbed through magazines or chatted up stylists as they spread bleach on strands of hair and wrapped them in foil. I sat under the hot dryer trying to breathe past the cutting odor of ammonia. Most stylists pushed for a dual process, which first required dying my darker brown hair a lighter brown shade. If I were in a lavish mood, I might concede. Normally, not, lest I be required to return to undergo this arduous process again even sooner. My streaks generally turned an ashy color, not the honey tone I envisioned, prompting me to try one stylist after another.

But wearing Gertrude, I no longer needed to fluff up my hair with my fingers or comb them through the back to cover a bare spot. When I passed a mirror, I marveled at what I saw on top of my head. For the first time in my life, I glimpsed the sense of assurance that comes with good hair.

I've always wished for thicker hair. This is a higher price than I ever wanted to pay.

Radiation started out as a nap on a hard surface. A machine circled my body, aiming a laser beam from different angles, supposedly to minimize burning the surface. I lay as still as I could so the beam would hit its precise target. I listened to Rod Stewart and memorized the lyrics to "As Time Goes By."

Dr. Forman, whom I saw once a week, was pleased with my progress.

"Fast-growing tumors shrink fast, though the shrinkage of cancerous masses can lag behind the death of cells, or apoptosis," he said.

"Get 'em," I said. I relished hearing him talk about killing cancer cells.

"Radiation is like shooting fish in a barrel," he said.

Before long, the skin around my vagina grew pinker. I could not only feel it, I could see it because chemo had also sent my pubic hair on a hike. I developed a bladder infection, diarrhea and vaginal discharge. After two and a half weeks, I complained to Dr. Forman. He examined me.

"Hmmm," he said from between my legs. "Your labia are receiving more radiation than I'd like. I'll adjust the beam. Your vagina is lined with glands. Radiation can increase mucus production by those glands. I'm not concerned about the discharge. It isn't foul-smelling."

Someone should have come up with a better word for the female orifice. Vagina sounds crude and threatening. That short "a" creeping in after a sneaky "v" and trailed by the whining, long "i." Words like nightingale or lily or martini have a softer, gentler ring. I would prefer to have had my doctor discussing my nightingale.

For much of my less-than-promiscuous life, I dropped my voice to utter the word vagina and its correlatives. "Cunt" was no better and contained a tinge of insult. "Clitoris" was another embarrassment, especially for such a handy little device. (I wasn't anti-feminist in my distaste for certain anatomical terms. "Penis" and "testicle" could also stand some improving.)

Eve Ensler liberated me. Several years before, I read in *The New York Times* that Ensler would soon stop performing her one-person play, *The Vagina Monologues*. I made a special trip to New York to see one of her last performances. Guiding me into the theater, an usher wore a badge that read "Vagina Bob." As he seated me, I said, "Thanks, Bob." Bob wasn't his name, he said. I'd understand after watching. The play was remarkable. I was knocked out by the courage the playwright/actor showed and by her compassion for women who had been sexually violated. Bob turned out to be someone Eve talked about in the play: a vulva connoisseur who appreciated, even worshipped, the female organ and to whom Ensler accorded hero status. On the way out, I noticed that all the male ushers wore Vagina Bob badges.

Thanks to Eve, aptly named for the source of the First Vagina, I became more grateful for my own female orifice and more comfortable mentioning it. After seeing the play, I began to pronounce all three syllables out loud, with appropriate emphasis, almost as unselfconsciously as I might say "apple tree." Still, discussing my tortured vagina with a cute fifty-something doctor I hardly knew, spread-eagled on an examining table, was a challenge. (I am tempted to say "stretch.")

Dr. Forman was slender with wavy, dark hair just beginning to fleck with grey. He was a friend of friends, someone I might run into at a party or restaurant. We should be talking over cocktails about the terroir or the notes of nutmeg in the wine we were sipping. We should be discussing the coral reefs we viewed while scuba diving in the Caymans. We should be toasting the Detroit Pistons recent win. He should be admiring the cut of my dress, the sparkle of my earrings. Not looking up my vagina. No less sniffing it.

At least I didn't smell, I thought. Amazing, in the face of death, the things you can still care about.

"There's some irritation in the back of your anus."

Anus? Another mortifying word. Was there no end to the indignities?

"The radiation beam is hitting that spot. Nothing to worry about."

"I'm having a problem with flatulence," I said. At that point, why not share another degradation? Fortunately, I didn't demonstrate it.

Dr. Forman stood up and snapped off his rubber gloves. "Another radiation side-effect," he said. "Between chemo and radiation, your gastro-intestinal tract is sensitive. Try Gas-X."

I developed a cough. Immediate thought: lung cancer. I called Dr. Malone. More likely a reaction to chemo, he said. My tongue, fingertips and toes started to tingle and turn numb.

Neuropathy, he said. Another chemo reaction. My diarrhea raged on. Probably from radiation, he said. My vagina continued to burn.

At our next appointment with my radiologist, Burton said, "Suzy is in so much pain already. I don't know how she can take any more."

Dr. Forman nodded. "I understand," he said. "Today is Wednesday. We can give you a little time to heal. We'll resume Monday. Five days off won't compromise your treatment."

If I hadn't been so sore, I would have leapt up and flung my arms around him. Instead I fell back on the table, clasped my hands over my chest and said, "Thank you, Lord."

We spent the time up north. I was overjoyed to discover that every day my crotch hurt a little less. On Sunday, as we headed home for more CT scans, my spirits collapsed.

I was sipping barium sulfate when David called.

"How ya doin', Mom?"

"Don't ask."

When David was a teenager, I tried to discourage his fondness for profanity. Swearing is lazy. It's sloppy. It's disrespectful, I said. When the foul language continued, I gave up trying to correct him. Prude that I once was, I decided it was better to hear four-letter words from my son than not to hear from him at all. Or to keep criticizing him.

"I remember a line from *Pulp Fiction*," David said. "In the movie, Marcellus Wallace has just been screwed in the ass. His friend asks how he's feeling. He says, 'I'm a long fucking way from alright.'"

I said, "I couldn't have put it better."

I pray my poor, little vagina has recovered enough in five days to tolerate the rest of radiation. I pray the CT scans show signs that radiation and chemo are working. I'm keeping God very busy with all these prayers.

CHAPTER 10

All That Really Matters

Ring the bells that still can ring. Forget your perfect offering. There is a crack in everything. That's how the light gets in.

—Leonard Cohen, "Anthem"

"HEALING IS ABOUT aligning your mental, emotional and nutritional relationships," Dr. Thomas said.

When you have cancer, you seek out all sorts of experts. Dr. Thomas was a multi-purpose expert—an M.D., a psychologist and a pharmacologist. He was also a cancer survivor who worked with cancer patients, one of whom recommended him to me. Three months into my saga, I called him.

Dr. Thomas wanted me to take lengthy psychological tests, to fast for a glucose test, to send for kits to check my stool, urine and blood. I would request these on the Internet, take delivery, poop or pee as directed, call Airborne Express for a pickup. His services would cost $10,000. I could read more about his approach on his website.

Dr. Thomas' credentials were impressive. But merely thinking about his program tired me. I barely had strength to stagger to the toilet, which I was doing with distressing frequency, no less answer dozens of questions and fill out reams of forms and align my mental, emotional and nutritional relationships. And for ten grand, if I failed to follow any instruction, I'd feel guilty and unaligned.

Also, I had assigned myself a project. Chemo affects everyone differently. I have girlfriends who continued to work at the office or walk for miles while in treatment. I needed to rest and was fortunate that I could. Since I was in bed so often, I decided to accomplish something I had long wanted to do but never found the time—a legacy to my sons.

Over the years I had kept journals, mostly on sleepless nights—one benefit of insomnia, along with sometimes catching Charlie Rose or finding time to edit my closet. I took these raggedy little books out of the bottom drawer of a file cabinet and searched for notes I had written about my sons as they were growing up. Since I had jotted their names in the margin when I wrote about them, I easily spotted those references. I typed anecdotes about David and Andy into separate files in my laptop computer. I wanted to give each of my sons his own journal, a record of his life through his mother's eyes.

Leaning against king-sized pillows, laptop propped on a bed table, I copied parts I had once handwritten. As I typed each one, I relived the feelings. I felt the anguish I'd experienced when David, at ten, came home with a scraped and bloodied face. He had fallen off his skateboard while attempting to ride holding on to the motorbike of the boy next door, also named David. (Next-door David was already on probation for egging our house on Halloween.) I felt awe recalling how Andy, at five, fell and broke his leg his first time down a ski slope and never cried. As a tear slalomed down my cheek, I realized he was braver at five than I was at sixty. I remembered what an anxious mother I was. Like little pack mules lumbering through time, my journals carried the burden of my worries.

Burton also came up with a project to help take his mind off our troubles. Once a week, he volunteered at lunchtime at Rodgers Academy, an ROTC-based, public high school in Detroit. An avid photographer, Burton started a photography club. Whether due to my husband's charisma or expertise or to the pizzas he always brought with him, club members showed up faithfully. Burton gave all his students point-and-shoot cameras and showed them how to use them. When he discovered that the school had not had a yearbook for ten years, he organized the club to produce one.

I had a few weeks to finish my sons' journals in time for Chanukah. If I spent what little energy I had completing Dr. Thomas' requirements, I would never meet my deadline. Besides, I was already taking supplements and monitoring my diet. I had talked with a couple of psychologists and continued speaking to my energy healer.

One lesson I was learning in my struggle with cancer: to put my needs first. I left a message for Dr. Thomas. I wasn't ready to work with him.

Compiling the boys' journals, I see how much time and energy I wasted worrying. Over the years, I worried about money, about my career, about the kids' safety and their grades. Most of what I worried about turned out fine. One lesson I hope I learn from my health problems is to let go of worry and trust that God will take care of all of us. This is a tough way to learn.

I was blessed with talented and accomplished girlfriends. One night in October, five of them joined me for dinner. Undergoing radiation as well as chemo, I felt neither talented nor accomplished. It was hard to believe I used to keep up with this lively group of women. But I was grateful for the company.

Brenda, my fashion maven/wig consultant/peace activist, wore a miniskirt, a tank top, opaque tights and Ugg boots. She owned a wardrobe of Uggs. She suffered problems with her feet stemming from many years in the fashion industry spent prancing around New York, Paris and Milan in high heels. Beth wore faded jeans. A renowned architectural photographer for national magazines, Beth was my partner when I was a regional design editor for *Better Homes and Gardens*. As confident as she was behind a lens, she was insecure about the way she dressed. When we worked together, she often asked my advice about what to wear. (I, no longer current, in turn asked Brenda.) Peggy wore a fringed, pastel jacket that was probably Chanel. She was clever about buying such extravagances on sale. Peggy was an advertising whiz, a vice president of *Condé Nast* magazines. Shelley wore a big, sparkly watch and a tight-fitting black leather jacket that showed off her enviable curves. She and her husband had developed and grown a successful optical chain. A bank owner and retired interior designer, Sandy accessorized a green print tunic with dark metal bangle bracelets. The tunic might have been from Bergdorf's or TJ Maxx; the bracelets were set with pave diamonds that could have been rose cut real stones or paste—Sandy was not a snob about provenance.

One of the nice parts of living for years in the same city is having your friends' kids become your kids' friends. Sandy's son Seth's vacation home was two doors from Andy's in northern Michigan. Peggy's son Josh, a real-estate investor in Chicago, grew up with David and Andy and remained one of their best pals. Shelley's daughter Jessica, a stand-up comedian in L.A., went to high school with Andy. One of the saddest parts of living in a shrinking city is the departure of much of the next generation. We felt lucky our sons were still in Detroit.

My girlfriends were in their fifties, younger than I, though not drastically. They looked great and vibrant. Some had had a little non-genetic help. I had avoided cosmetic procedures. Now the thought of volunteering for any more needles or knives seemed incomprehensible.

We sat in the library, sipping cabernet or vodka. We devoured hummus, tabouleh and dry-rubbed spareribs from Phoenicia in Birmingham, arguably one of the finer Lebanese restaurants anywhere. As much as I adored their ribs, in my quest to eat healthier, I hadn't indulged since I was diagnosed. They tasted salty, crunchy, chewy and decadent, especially dipped into barbeque sauce with just the right kick.

Although the significance of the day had escaped the rest of us, Brenda told us it was *Simchat* Torah. She reminded us that the Jewish holiday celebrates the end of the annual cycle of public Torah readings and the beginning of a new cycle. On *Simchat* Torah, Hebrew for "rejoicing in the law," the last verses of Deuteronomy are read, followed by the first verses of Genesis.

Brenda led us in an informal service. We lit candles, sang songs and recited blessings. Concluding our service, Brenda said, "*Simchat* Torah reminds us that life has ends and beginnings. Let's pray it means a quick end to Suzy's treatment and the beginning of her new life, free of cancer."

"Amen, sister," I said.

After, the conversation turned to girl talk. Beth brought up the subject of chemical facial peels and how long it takes to recover from them. Brenda said she had seen a new type of facelift featured on TV. Strings were implanted into your cheeks and tightened to lift your jowls.

I decided to share a lesson in humility. "I can't worry about sagging skin," I said. "Right now all I want is to control my bowels. Cancer has knocked my ego flat. Being homebound. Looking like a ghost. Not even being able to plan lunch because doctors' appointments take precedence and I don't know how I'll feel from day to day. Take it from me. All that matters is a healthy body."

Four shiny, well-cut, newly-colored heads and a silver/grey one bobbed up and down. "You are so right," they chorused.

I smiled, gratified that my message had gotten through.

Sandy said, "Emmes," Hebrew for truth.

"Thanks for reminding us," Beth said.

"I learn so much from you," Shelley said.

Peggy nodded gravely. "We need to be less concerned about our looks."

Brenda put her hand on my knee. "You're so brave," she said. "You give me courage to work for interfaith peace among hostile groups."

I looked at Brenda and shook my head. "You chose your fight," I said.

Minutes later, we heard Burton walk through the back door. It was late. My girlfriends started gathering their things.

Shelley pulled a business card from her oversized black leather Chanel bag. "Wait," she said, tossing her wavy, black mane. "I almost forgot. I've got to give you all something important. The number of my vein-stripping doctor."

Having studied French for five years, I can't resist throwing an occasional *bon mot*, or French word, into a sentence. And sometimes launching the whole sentence. I'm especially fond of a saying introduced by French novelist/journalist/critic Jean-Baptiste Alphonse Karr in the journal he produced in the mid-1800s.

"Plus ça change, plus c'est la même chose," I said. The more things change, the more they remain the same.

When Shelley produced the number for her vein-stripping doctor, my girlfriends all took out their pens.

Rebekka's hands skimmed the blanket she had wrapped around me. "Cancer invites you to grow," she said. "It moved you to a deeper place, a place you wouldn't have gotten without it, a place of total love. Bless your diagnosis."

I lay still and tried to dredge up gratitude for my lack of energy and inflamed vagina and uncertain prospects. I found not a cell, not an atom, not the nucleus of an atom of gratitude. Fear stabbed me in the stomach and twisted the knife.

"I can't bless it," I wailed. "This is too hard."

Rebekka was usually perceptive, I thought, but this time she was off her rocker. I'd like to see her bless her fried vagina.

"Physical and emotional torture is not my idea of total love."

"Detach from the self who is a writer or wife or mother or cancer patient. Those roles belong to the physical realm. They're not real in an eternal sense. When you detach from them, you can marvel at how sacred and glorious you are. If you are joyful, feel it. If you're tired, rest. You're learning to stay in the moment, to bring quality to each experience." Rebekka's hands alighted on my chest and my pelvis.

I remained doubtful.

"Let me tell you a Buddhist story," she said. "A tiger chases a man to the edge of a cliff. There the man sees a bush with one plump, ripe berry hanging from it. With the tiger bearing down on him, the man stops to enjoy that berry."

"Then what?"

"The story ends there."

Burton also had someone who helped give him perspective. Soon after I got sick, he began studying with an Orthodox rabbi. Although we were both Reformed Jews, Burton appreciated the rabbi's scholarship. He met with Rabbi Cohen twice a week and drew comfort from their conversations. In the early mornings, Burton read prayer books and the Torah.

I remained perplexed about Rebekka's Buddhist story. I said to Burton, "There is no way I could have enjoyed that berry."

Burton said, "I've been reading about the sacrifices God required of our ancestors. It's giving me insight into our struggle. God wants us to sacrifice some coping behaviors we think we need and to trust Him."

"What coping behaviors?"

"In my case, my desire to control the outcome. In yours, negative thinking. It's like God is saying, 'My shoulders are broad. I'll take care of you.' This illness is a way for both of us to become closer to God. I hope we get it right this time."

I shook my head. "My faith is being tested. I'm flunking."

A friend flew us up north for the weekend. When the plane taxied to a stop, I raced to the bathroom to rub numbing cream on my scalded vagina. I wasn't there when the pilot unloaded the plane.

Later, at our farmhouse, I looked for my wig.

"Have you seen Gertrude?" I asked Burton.

"No. Where was she?"

"On the plane."

"In what?"

"A white plastic bag."

"What was on the bag?"

"Nothing," I said. Ice froze my stomach. "It was a kitchen trash bag."

Burton refrained from observing that a kitchen trash bag was a really stupid place to put an expensive wig. "Call the airport," he said.

I explained the problem to the receptionist. She checked with the pilot. No one noticed a plain white plastic bag. It could have been considered garbage and thrown out, she said.

I fought for breath.

"I know this is an inconvenience, but could you please ask someone to check the dumpster?"

"It's dark and raining."

"I'm fighting cancer. That wig is really important to me."

Her voice softened. "I'll talk to the ground crew."

Minutes later, she called back. "I'm so sorry."

Panic flooded my chest. My heart pounded. I lay on my bed in the dark. It's only a wig, I scolded myself. It's not your life. I thought about some of the advice I'd received. Rebekka said bless my diagnosis. What a load of crap. Donna said observe my thoughts. I'm observing alright. Observing terror. My wig had taken two weeks to make and had cost enough to feed a family for a month. How could I have been so careless?

I shoved my mind back to a visit I made five years before. I traveled to the Deepak Chopra Center to work with self-help guru Debbie Ford. It was soon after Burton and I had attended our couples program and had begun to work on resolving our problems. Debbie's book *The Dark Side of the Light Chasers* had shown me a way to begin healing. I had made a pilgrimage to La Jolla to attend one of her sessions. The last exercise Debbie gave my group that weekend was to compile a gratitude list. Twenty things for which we were thankful. "If you do this every day, it will change your life," Debbie said. I did, in writing at first. Then, through prayer. It had helped. But thrashing on my bed, I was fresh out of gratitude. I couldn't focus on anything but how stupid I had been.

Brenda had helped create Gertrude. She'd understand. I picked up the phone. "I'm freaking out," I wailed. "I know I'm being a baby."

"Don't be so hard on yourself," Brenda said. "That wig is your life raft in a sea of uncertainty. Losing a wig isn't losing your will to live. Maybe there's a reason you lost it. Maybe you need to face your feelings about what you're going through."

Brenda kept talking, calmly, reasonably. Not once did she remind me that she had recommended getting two wigs. She stayed on the phone until my gasping subsided. Hanging up, I thought about what she'd said. I had been careening back and forth between trying hard not to worry and trying equally hard to be brave. I had screwed the cap on my emotions as if they were an old bottle of rubber cement. My feelings were clogged and hardened in the bottom.

Brenda was right. I needed a serious cry. I gave in.

The next day, the wig still hadn't shown up. Panic squeezed my lungs again. Cara, a friend who survived breast cancer, called. I told her how I'd come unraveled about my wig. She told me about a psychologist who treated people for anxiety disorders and worked with cancer patients.

Back in Detroit, I wore a cotton cap to the office of Dr. Daitch. "I'm not surprised," she said. "That wig was one of the only things under your control right now."

She understood. She got it. A tiny crack opened in my clogged chest.

"When we can't fix a problem, the best we can do is to acknowledge our feelings," Dr. Daitch said. She gave me an exercise in what she called mindfulness.

"Close your eyes. Ask yourself: What am I feeling right now? Anger? Rage? Grief?"

"Terror."

"Tell yourself, I am my terror. Then take a deep breath and say, I breathe through my terror. I am more than my terror."

I repeated the exercise a few times. By the time I left, I could breathe again.

Brenda's ability to talk me down, Cara's understanding, Dr. Daitch's perspective—I still hadn't connected the dots. I didn't see that they were part of a greater whole. I didn't perceive how remarkable it was that when I needed something, it was revealed. The pattern the dots make is only visible in retrospect, looking back. With backward eyes.

When the diagnosis is cancer, people go out of their way to help. Late that afternoon, the airport receptionist called. The ground crew searched through the dumpster in daylight, she said. They spotted the white bag.

Gertrude was found.

One Indian-summer weekend up north, I sat in my favorite spot, on our porch swing. I skimmed one of my old journals for excerpts on David and Andy. The project had helped take my mind off how tired I was from chemo and how sore from radiation. I sat in my usual position, leaning against one arm of the swing, shoes off, legs extended on the seat.

Tucked against my pelvis, my laptop computer warmed a part of my body that had recently been cut, eviscerated and radiated. Feels good, I thought. Suddenly I grew cold. I always sat the same way, with my back against the arm of the swing. The western afternoon sun shone on my shoulders. The computer pressed more firmly against my left side due to the slant of the swing.

I thought about the cancer that had invaded my pelvis. By the time my tumor was discovered, it had destroyed ninety percent of the left side of my pelvic bone, sixty percent of the right.

I stood up, walked into the house, and propped my computer on a table.

Later, I asked my allopathic doctors if electromagnetic energy could have caused or worsened my cancer. Unlikely, they said. But several months after, I heard about an urologist who had lectured in Detroit. He claimed that an alarming percentage of his prostate cancer patients worked with laptop computers in their laps.

I never did again, and when I see others doing so, I pester them about it.

Denise and Andrei, two of my radiation technicians, were friendly but professional. They chatted with me before and after treatment. I learned that Andrei, a Russian immigrant, hated the countryside and resented the high price of gas, then about $1.88 for a gallon of regular. Denise, with the pins on her lapel, loved northern Michigan and baked delicious Toll House cookies, some of which she had brought me. But as the effects of radiation ganged up on me, I began to regard my likable technicians as stealth torturers.

The antibiotics I took for my bladder infection worsened my vaginal infection. My vagina bled from irritation. My urethra stung as though on fire when I peed. Due to my continuing bladder infection, I had to pee constantly.

Dr. Mike, my regular gynecologist who months ago had met me in his office at 7 a.m. to perform my D&C, checked in often. When I first started chemo, he called to see if I had received a flu shot. With my immune system compromised by chemo, I was more susceptible, he said. "I'm coming over to give you a flu shot," he insisted and showed up at our door within the hour.

In the midst of my radiation woes, Dr. Mike called again. How was I doing?

"Crappy."

"Use anything that helps." He suggested AnaMantle cream, which contained Xylocaine and a steroid for my burning, bleeding vaginal tissue. And Gynazole for my bladder infection.

"Whatever you do, stick with aggressive treatment," he said. "This is like playing defense in football. The first quarter isn't so tough. The hard part comes later, when you're beaten up and can barely breathe. That's when you need the internal fire to make your body do what it doesn't want to do."

"I'm feeling fire alright, but at the wrong end."

To alleviate the pain when I peed, he suggested filling the bathtub with water and sitting in it to urinate, thus diluting the acid. I was reluctant to pee in my tub. It would take too long to fill the tub, and I didn't want to keep cleaning it.

I said to Burton, "Maybe there's some plastic container I could put in the tub and fill with water."

"I'm on it," he said and raced to the garage.

Home Depot was fifteen minutes from our house. Burton returned in less than half an hour. He ran into the house and thrust out a grey, flexible plastic bin about two feet square with low, curved sides. "For mixing cement," he said. "Will it work?"

Having held my urine for his return, I sped to the bathroom, shoved the bin under the tub faucet and jerked the handles for hot and cold water. I climbed out of my terrycloth capris and old-lady underpants, stepped into the tub, lowered my butt into warm water, and peed.

Burton had followed me into the bathroom. He bit his lip and looked at me with the breath-stopping focus with which he would watch a 30-foot putt curve toward the hole and hesitate on the rim.

"Well?"

"Better." I smiled up at him from the tub. "Bless you."

He pumped his fist. "Hoo-ah."

As long as I was home when I needed to pee, sitting in the water-filled cement container helped considerably. When I was out, the pain remained searing.

The redness and burning continued. I slathered cream on my burned anus and labia and on my itching vagina. I tried numbing sprays. Whenever possible, I left off my underpants. I felt like I was suffering the Egyptian plagues. Frogs, my burned rectum. Lice, my bladder infection. Locusts, candida. Pestilence, boils and hail stones were next.

I wrote in my journal: *Let my cancer go.*

CHAPTER 11

Superman, Fallen

I called on God from a narrow place; God answered from a wide expanse.

—from **Psalm 118**

IT WAS 7:30 a.m. The morning after my CT scans, the ring awakened us.

"Hello?" I said, still groggy.

"This is Dr. Forman. I'm on my way out of town, but I wanted you to know."

I snapped to attention. Dr. Forman had never called me before. He sounded upbeat. You can tell when someone is smiling on the other end of a phone. You can hear it in his inflection, in the tone of his voice.

"What?" I said, squeezing the receiver.

"I looked at your scans this morning," he said. "Your brain and chest are clear. The lesions in your pelvic bone are about eighty percent gone. Some reossification is already occurring. This is good news."

My heart swelled. I caught my breath. "Thank you," I exclaimed. "Tell Burton."

Burton must have been unusually tired because he still lay in bed. As I handed him the phone, a little crack of hope began forming in the shell around my heart.

Burton has been through a lot. He started working as a newsboy at age nine, the year his father, Simon, a family doctor, was sent to a tuberculosis clinic in Saranac Lake, New York. He died there two years later of what proved to be a misdiagnosed pancreatic disease. The day his father died, Burton and his sisters sat through two showings of *Gone with the Wind* before someone came to pick them up. As much as he loves movies, he has not been able to watch that one again. To support her son and two daughters, Burton's widowed mother, Edith, went to work as a high-school math teacher. Family and friends told Burton he had to be "the man of the house." To make money, he shoveled snow, whitewashed basements for a building company and developed a bagel route. He struggled academically, skipping school when he could, staying home to watch TV. Not knowing he had ADD, Burton saw himself as "lazy and stupid". He bounced between high schools. Still, he grew up to build a successful real-estate company and to run numerous charitable and civic boards. He supported my publishing a book about our marriage problems, despite his personal embarrassment, because he thought we could help others. In other words, Burton is a strong man.

The call we received that morning was the first real evidence that all the research Burton had done, all the medical decisions he'd made, all the suffering I had endured seemed to be working. It was the first real moment in almost three months that we sensed we might win the chance to meet all of our grandchildren together. We might get to play in more mixed member/guest golf tournaments and savor more sunsets in Florida. We might have a future. After talking to Dr. Forman, my strong husband wiped his eyes with the back of a hand so big I had called it a paw. He drew me to him. We lay in bed with our separate thoughts, feeling each other's warmth, too moved to speak.

Responses to cancer treatment differ for everyone. However far medical science has progressed, there is still the unknown. Doctors predict which protocol is likely to be most effective, but there are no guarantees. I had endured weeks of tough treatment with no certainty that the process would work. From the lilt in my doctor's voice, from his taking the time to call right away, I knew he shared my relief. Moments like this, I realized, not only kept patients and their loved ones going. They kept doctors going, too.

October 15, 2004. I drew stars across the top of the page in my journal.

Radiation is based on quantum physics. Packets of energy are delivered in wave form through a proton beam. The beam consists of volts of electrons which can be shaped for greater accuracy. A tumor is targeted from several angles to minimize the effects on skin and other healthy tissue. Since I underwent radiation, techniques have become even more precise.

The proton beam damages the DNA (the molecules inside cells that carry and pass on genetic information) of whatever cells it targets. Those cells deteriorate. Some are killed immediately; some are damaged and die over time. Some are damaged but can repair themselves; some can escape unharmed. The more treatments, the better the chance of killing all the cancerous cells.

Theoretically, proton-beam radiation spares healthy tissue. Realistically, by week number five, my vagina was so fried that I begged for relief. Dr. Forman had agreed to give me three days off, plus a weekend. Five days free from radiation had sped by. My crotch had healed enough that it no longer felt scorched, merely tender.

Burton and I were back in Dr. Forman's office. Dr. Forman studied my latest abdominal and pelvic CT scans on his computer screen.

"The huge masses and extension into the muscle are gone," he said. "Your pelvic bone is healing. It's also encouraging that cancer doesn't appear to be growing anywhere else."

He looked up and smiled. "This is a helluva response."

I bit my lip. Burton choked back a sob.

I felt like I was back in fourth grade at Washington School in Royal Oak, Michigan and I had won a spelling bee, and Miss LaForge had peered at me through her frameless spectacles and called me her "little chickadee." Miss LaForge was one of my all-time favorite teachers.

Dreading the side effects of further radiation, I asked, "What if we stopped now?"

"The extent of your response indicates that your cancer is really sensitive. We want to keep it away as long and as permanently as possible. We know the optimum dosage. We're not there yet. If I didn't see progress, or the tumor had spread, I'd say forget it.

"Radiation effects are cumulative. I don't want to give you so much time off that the cancer starts growing again. The fact that you're feeling better gives you a sense of how the body can repair and heal.

"The only thing that hasn't significantly improved is the nodule in your thyroid. It appears to have reduced slightly, but the response is not as dramatic as in your pelvis."

"So radiation has been more effective than chemo?"

He drummed his index finger on his desk. "It appears so. I'm happy with what we've accomplished in a relatively short time. Considering what we're doing to you, your side effects could be worse."

I groaned.

"I know this is hard on you, Suzy. You can't make an omelet without breaking an egg. After surgery, radiation and chemo, chances are all the cancer is gone from your pelvis. Your side effects aren't likely to get much worse in the next few days."

"What about recurrence?"

"It's possible. I'm more concerned about other areas, like your lungs."

"Because my body produced one type of cancer, am I more likely than anyone else to get any other kind?"

"No."

I exhaled with relief.

"Four more days of burning pee," I said. "Somehow I'll tough them out."

Dr. Forman cocked an eyebrow. "It's not four. It's eight more treatments. 4,500 units of radiation, or rads, suffice for the area where your uterus and ovaries were removed. Your pelvic bone requires 6,000 rads."

"Eight?" I wailed. We had misunderstood the schedule. I was never very good at math. Especially now when it had to do with what felt like swarms of fire ants stinging my vagina. Tears welled up in my eyes. It was all I could do not to cry. I started to shake.

Burton took my hand. "Suzy's had so much pain already. I don't know how she can take eight more days," he said.

"A little more time off won't hurt our results." Dr. Forman said. "Today is Monday. We'll resume Wednesday."

Burton and I and headed out into the chilly air. I chanted: I am my pain. I breathe through my pain. I am more than my pain. There was no escape. Four chemos to go. Eight more days of a burning ass and stinging pee. " … A case of do or die." I'd know every damn word of the song *As Time Goes By* before I was done. But I had two more days to recover. I'd do my best to enjoy every second.

Be careful what you wish for, St. Teresa of Ávila warned. For years I had prayed to better stay in the moment. Yet another lesson I was learning the hard way.

"Don and I are chairing the annual Karmanos fund-raising dinner next May," my friend Jinny said on the phone. "We want you and Burt to be honorary chairs. It would mean so much to honor someone who was treated there. Please say you'll accept."

"Thank you for thinking of us. What would we have to do?"

"Take a table. Encourage friends to come. And say a few words."

I counted the months on my fingers.

"May is seven months away. What makes you think I'll even be here?"

"I asked your doctors."

"And?"

"And they promised you would."

Goose bumps rose on my arms. It was one thing to have my doctors seem optimistic with me. It was another to have them agree to put me in an official position which, if I didn't make it, could be bad publicity for the hospital. Normally I would ask Burton's opinion before accepting such a position; this time I had no doubt about how he'd feel.

"In that case, we're in," I said. "I'll have quite a story to tell."

During my final week of radiation, I went back to see Dr. Daitch. I was grateful to have someone to talk to whose job it was to listen to my complaints.

"I hate feeling sorry for myself. And having so little control."

"When events run counter-intuitive to how we're wired, we need to move to a place of stillness," she said. "Pause and ask yourself: At this moment, should I be proactive? Or should I trust?" Dr. D. sat in a big chair that made her small frame seem even smaller. She tapped a pencil against her hand.

"This illness is a blow to the part of you that cares about achievement and recognition and appearance. The challenge is to calm down and transcend your ego. If you don't fight a reaction, you can float through it. Physically, how do you feel at this moment?"

I surveyed my body, head to toe. "Okay."

"Keep going back to the moment. Tell yourself: Right now I'm brushing my teeth; I'm putting on my glasses; I'm getting in the car. Your brain needs to be occupied so it doesn't overwhelm you with terror. Keep your brain busy on the now."

On my way out of the office, I noticed an issue of *People*. Christopher Reeve was on the cover. I stopped, stared at the headline, and gasped. I picked up the magazine and flipped to the article. Until recently I'd kept track of how Brad and Angelina were getting along and who Jennifer Aniston's latest boyfriend was and other useless items of popular culture. Now,

I realized, I was so absorbed in my own problems I didn't even know Christopher Reeve had died a week ago.

As I trudged to the car, I thought about the grace with which Reeve had borne his paralysis. I thought about the courage he had shown. And about how hard his illness must have been on his ego. Superman, fallen.

I can still talk to my sons and hug my husband and kiss my granddaughter's head, I thought. And for the first time in a while, I cried for someone else. I cried for Christopher Reeve.

> *Five days since my last chemo. The steroids have worn off. I'm exhausted. My ass burns. My new theme song: "Rawhide."*
>
> *Cancer steals your confidence in the future. I look at other people as the healthy ones, the ones with enough energy to play golf or go to the office. They can take their grandkids to a park and not worry if they'll live to see them strong enough to hang from the monkey bars or brave enough to tackle the high slide. No one really knows if they'll be around tomorrow, but illness brings a new sense of vulnerability.*
>
> *I try not to think about the possibility that all this treatment won't kill every single bad cell.*

On October 30, I lay on the hard radiation table and prayed I would never, ever need pelvic radiation again. The machine finished its circuit around me, moving and stopping and buzzing, and retreated to its starting place overhead to the left. Denise, my technician, walked into the room. She was beaming.

"You did it," she said.

"Thank God it's over," I said. "You bake cookies better than people."

Denise laughed.

Four days later, my vagina had progressed from burning to merely itching. I never imagined I would feel grateful for an itching vagina.

Up north the weekend after radiation ended, Burton and I walked the two-track to and from the lake, about a half-mile each way. With every dip in the road, my husband took my arm to steady me. The sun shone brighter, the aspen leaves trembled more delicately than ever. Hundreds of Canada geese swam on the lake, honking loudly, discussing their fall travel plans.

It was toward the end of my three-week chemo cycle, so some of my energy had returned. I was pleased to make it both ways without pain in my groin. With the tumors removed, my pelvic-bone fracture was healing. I prayed the tumors were gone for good. As elated as I was to have finished radiation, I was nervous to have lost a key defense.

My bowels returned to normal. The itching and discharge in my vagina lessened each day. My respite did not last long. Soon I was back at Karmanos. Dr. Malone checked my blood and vital signs, declared me healthy enough to undergo my next chemo.

I complained about having so little pep.

"You are basically a healthy person being put through poison," he said. "By February, you should feel almost yourself again."

A miscommunication between the doctor and the lab held up the delivery of my chemo potion for a couple of hours. By the time I was finished, it was dark outside. Leaving the chemo ward, Burton put his arm around my shoulders. For the ump-teenth time in recent weeks, I marveled that this man, who a few years ago had been so emotionally and physically absent in our marriage, was so totally present now.

Since my previous book qualifies me as somewhat of a rela-tionship expert, I should add that I don't recommend cancer as a way of mending a broken marriage. I've seen as many hus-bands desert a wife facing a medical crisis as I have seen those who rally. I was just grateful that Burton belonged to the group of men who come through, who see the challenge, grit their teeth and fight. Who are men of valor.

"Four down. Two to go," Burton said. "We're almost there."

That night I experienced a nosebleed and diarrhea. The left side of my groin felt tender. I didn't mention it to Burton. He would ask if was worse or better than before. I didn't know. The tenderness worried me. I feared it meant that chemo wasn't working after all, or that cancer had returned. The amygdala is a small ganglion in our brain responsible for fear. My amygdala went on heightened alert.

I read for all kinds of reasons. For the story. For the love of language. For insight. For picking up odd facts. Usually, I read books that are recommended by people I respect. Once when I attended a writers' conference, an agent horrified most of the audience by declaring, "I can tell whether or not someone can write from the first page of a manuscript. Actually, I can tell from the first sentence." I thought the agent made sense. Since then I have learned to read the first page of a book that looks appealing. From those few words, I'll decide if this is an author with whom I want a relationship.

That night I read to distract myself, to give my overworked little amygdala a break. I picked up a book everyone was raving about, *The Kite Runner* by Khaled Hosseini. "I became what I am today at the age of twelve … " The story gripped me right away. I had never before so appreciated the power of a good book to help me escape.

Three days after chemo Burton planned to spend a night up north. I assured him I'd be fine. Reluctant to leave me alone, he asked Brenda to stay overnight.

Brenda and two more of my talented and accomplished girlfriends came for dinner. Hsaio-Ping was an Asian-American in the import/export business who grew prize-winning orchids in her spare time. Lila, of Lebanese descent, ran a medical supply company. Hsaio-Ping brought her rice steamer containing a delicious chicken soup flavored with wine, scallions and ginger.

"The Chinese, like the Jews, make chicken soup when someone is ill," she said. "It's guaranteed to make you well."

After dinner we sat in the library and drew from Brenda's deck of angel cards. The three cards we each picked seemed destined for us.

One of Brenda's cards was "Divine Inspiration." She saw it as encouragement to keep working for interfaith peace. Lila, then facing business challenges, received "Protection," featuring the Archangel Michael. "He's the patron saint of the warrior," she said. "He keeps showing up in my life." Hsaio-Ping and her husband had been working overtime to provide relief housing in third-world countries. "Balance" reminded her to pay attention to her personal life.

I received "Divine Timing": Walk through open doors. Learn from shut doors. You can't skip or rush the process. "Trust": Have faith that God and the angels are with you. They'll help you to trust yourself. And "Signs": Notice and trust the signs the angels bring you.

"Amazing," I said. I shook my head. "But I'm still worried."

Lila, who has a knack for getting to the point, said, "Suzy, what does God have to do for you? Show up on a magic carpet?"

Later that night, I lay in bed alone for the first time since I returned from surgery three months before. My groin again felt sore. I prayed the ache came from the walk I had taken with Burton earlier, or that it simply meant my bone was healing. Still, my limbs twitched; my heart pounded.

I padded barefoot down the stairs to our lower level. Brenda was staying in the guest room. The light was out.

I knocked on her door. "I'm sorry to bother you."

"That's why I'm here," she said. She came up to my bedroom with me, sat on my bed and held my hand.

"I know my healing is God's will," I wailed. "But I don't know what God's will is."

Brenda rubbed my hand and let me cry.

"Remember the cards you drew tonight?"

I nodded.

"Be patient. Trust that you are healing. Those were signs. God was speaking to you."

When my heart slowed and I could breathe again, I sent Brenda back to bed. I lay back down and thought about what Brenda had said. And about what Lila said. God would not appear on a flying carpet. He did not have to. His presence was clear in the cards I drew. That should be enough to let me sleep.

I can be remarkably short-sighted. I still didn't look back at all the other ways God had shown up in the past few weeks. But as for that night, Brenda was right. Her angel cards trumpeted a message I longed to hear. I just needed a little more faith.

Burton and I had hosted our family's Thanksgiving dinner for over thirty years. This fall, as my favorite holiday neared, I wondered how I'd have the strength to organize the celebration. Fortunately, Andy and Amy volunteered to give up their plans to visit Amy's parents in Atlanta and to stay home and take over. Amy's mom, dad and sister all joined us in Michigan. I was especially grateful not to be in charge on Thanksgiving morning. Sautéeing onions and mushrooms in olive oil, I felt so weak that I collapsed back in bed. Burton finished making the stuffing and took care of roasting the turkey.

Andy roasted a turkey, too. Before dinner, we gathered in Andy and Amy's kitchen, mouths watering from the aroma of sage, rosemary and thyme. "Let's see whose tastes better," Andy said.

Two glistening, browned turkeys rested on cutting boards on the granite-topped island. Burton carved one; Andy, the other. Burton removes the breast meat and cuts down, then transfers the uniform slices to a platter. He taught this method to Andy. The rest of us watched this culinary display, urging them to expedite. The minute knives were removed, we dove in to the scraps. Using our fingers, we chomped on warm, dripping bites of light and dark meat. A chorus of "mmms" arose.

Andy said, "Mine's better—right, Mom? It's juicier."

The men in our family are competitive. They challenge each other to basketball games. They make bets as to who can give the closest estimate for arcane questions like what is the current minimum wage and what big city has the highest rate of poverty. (Unfortunately we all knew the last answer.) If there's no official athletic missile present, they throw stones or pine cones at tree trunks to see whose aim is better. Their competitive endeavors are always accompanied by boasts about their respective prowess. A Ping-Pong match between the three of them makes the annual U OF M/Ohio State football game look like a love fest.

Raising two boys, I have learned diplomacy. Mothers master this skill. Gifts, compliments, time spent—all must be equal. There ought to be a job requirement that the U.S. Secretary of State first serve as a mom. The world would be a more peaceful place.

As lackluster as I felt, I was lucid enough not to be dragged into a trap. "Both turkeys are delicious," I said. "If yours is juicier than ours, it's because it didn't travel."

Amy set the dining-room table with crystal and floral china. I had long since stopped using my best tableware on Thanksgiving because it had to be washed by hand and kitchen help was scarce and costly. I admire hosts who can leave dirty dishes stacked on the counter, or in the oven, to be attacked the next day. I wasn't one of them. I can't bear to watch gravy congeal. But Amy's table looked beautiful.

Turkey, cranberry sauce, mashed sweet potatoes, green bean and mushroom casserole—all were as delicious as ever. David and I normally share the neck, but this year we each got one of our own. We nibbled away at the tender, salty meat between the small bones. The turkey neck is David's and my favorite part, one which we are pleased to observe goes unappreciated by the rest of the family each year.

As healthy as my appetite was, I still felt exhausted. After dinner I slumped in my chair. "I'm sorry I don't have the strength to help," I said.

"Next year you will," Amy's mom said. I wished I felt as confident as Carol sounded.

We were back at our son's house the next night. Andy invited me to watch him give Alexis a bath. He filled a plastic container with a few inches of warm water, tested the temperature with his elbow, then lowered his daughter's small, pink body into the water. He cradled her head in one hand. Both of our boys have Burton's big hands.

Andy dipped a washcloth into the warm water and squeezed it over Alexis several times. He bent down and blew into her belly, making a sputtering sound and causing her lips to curve in a smile. He rubbed baby shampoo on her hair and pulled it into a little peak as I once did with him. Rinsing the shampoo with cupfuls of water, he held her head back with as much care and patience as he would bring to studying the numbers of a real-estate deal.

I listened to small, splashing sounds, inhaled the sweet smell of shampoo and wondered where my big, brawny son developed such delicate skill. I thought about how lucky my granddaughter was to have such a tender, caring father.

I whispered, "This is one of the most beautiful things I've ever seen."

Andy patted Alexis dry, wrapped her in a towel and cradled her in his arms. Holding her dark, damp head next to his cheek, he said, "You know what I think, Mom? As a child, you take four or five years to develop real love for your parents. When you meet the person you marry, you take four or five months to fall in love. When you have a baby, love is instant."

Cancer heightens your awareness. You know in every fiber and cell that certain times will not come again. You stop and savor moments that might otherwise slip by, unnoticed. Cancer makes you remember.

Dr. Forman studied the dark image of my latest CT scan. He looked up from his computer screen and nodded. "Your massive tumor involvement is gone. Your pelvic bone is remarkably improved. There is no visible tumor left."

Burton and I exhaled. Tears welled up in both our eyes. I had spent so many weeks stalked by worry, so many days dragging my raw ass around in pain and exhaustion. Now, with one glorious apparition on an impartial computer monitor—a machine that didn't care whether I lived or died or had a granddaughter with navy blue eyes or a marriage that had also suffered a narrow escape—everything I'd endured in the past few months suddenly seemed worthwhile.

My skin flushed warm. My lungs filled with air. What a difference thirty seconds made.

I stood up and walked over to the computer. "Can you show me my first x-ray?"

Dr. Forman tapped on his keyboard and pulled up a second image. "This is your original scan," he said. A massive, white shape obliterated the left side of my pelvis and much of the right. "Those white areas are tumor." He split the screen so I could compare the old and new images. The difference was literally black-and-white.

"Oh my God," I said. My knees started to shake. "Did I see this before?"

"You did."

"I'm glad I didn't know what I was looking at."

Driving home in the car, I asked Burton if he had understood how frightening my first pelvic scan was.

He drummed his thumbs on the steering wheel. "I understood," he said. "It gave me some pretty rough nights, especially when everyone had a different idea about the protocol. I felt better when all the doctors finally agreed. Dr. Ruckdeschel said there was an eighty percent chance the treatment would work. I decided to believe him."

Burton took my hand and kissed my fingertips. "We've been through some rough months," he said. "Thank God they're paying off."

CHAPTER **12**

Backward Eyes

*My friend Sophie calls it coincidence, and Mr.
Simpless, my parson friend, calls it Grace. He
thinks that if one cares deeply about someone or
something new, one throws a kind of energy out
into the world, and "fruitfulness" is drawn in.*

—**Mary Ann Shaffer and Annie Barrows,** *The
Guernsey Literary and Potato Peel Pie Society*

I STOPPED FOR a salad at Steve's Deli and sat next to
a mother and daughter. The mother looked to be in her early
eighties; the daughter, about my age. I envied their relaxed conversation. It had been several years since my mother and I had
gone out to lunch.

Mom remained reclusive. Although we spoke most days, I
hadn't visited in over three months. I had recovered from surgery and radiation and would soon finish chemo. It was time to
see my mother again.

That afternoon I lay on Rebekka's table. Hands gliding above
me, she said, "You seem anxious."

"I'm about to visit my mother."

"It feels like your mother is carrying a laundry load on her
head and you keep sticking your head under it," she said. "Your
mother chose her own laundry. You don't need to carry it."

That evening I picked up moo shu chicken for me and egg foo young for Mom—plain, the way she liked it, though nothing brought her much pleasure anymore. I trudged past several elderly people sitting and chatting in the lobby, signed in, rode the elevator to seven and walked to Mom's door. I took a deep breath and turned the knob.

Aside from the emotional strain of visiting my mother, there were physical constraints. We had no privacy. Mom's hearing had deteriorated; I had to speak forcefully. Meaningful conversations do not lend themselves to a loud delivery, especially with an aide in the next room. I was reluctant to let the aide leave in case Mom needed to use the toilet, which she often did. I lacked the strength and skill to help her on or off. Aides had a way of being hard to reach once they left the apartment. I wasn't confident I could contact them in an emergency. When I had let them take breaks, there had been times I had been unable to reach them. When they returned, they had claimed problems with their cell phones.

I ate and Mom nibbled at dinner. I rinsed the dishes and we worked a crossword puzzle Mom had saved from the *Detroit Free Press*. The puzzle gave us a congenial way to spend time and to share an activity we both enjoyed. It gave each of us a chance to see that Mom still had some mental acuity. When there was an answer I thought she might know, I waited to see if she came up with it. One clue in that night's puzzle was: The Godfather. I was happy to hear Mom say, "Marlon." It was early in the week so the puzzle was relatively easy, and we finished it. I signed it with Mom's initials and mine, two happy faces and two stars. (To this day, though Mom is no longer around, whenever I master a crossword puzzle, I continue to sign it with both of our initials. It remains my personal tribute to my once-smart and curious mother.)

"We did it," I said, smacking the table with my fist.

Mom said, as she always did, "It was mostly you."

I shook my head. "You got Marlon."

Mom was glad to see me. She did not comment on how long it had been. I didn't mention how lonely she must be, stuck in her apartment. That was her laundry.

If anyone ever had the right to complain, Mom did. One decision, intended to enhance her so-called golden years, ended her ability to do most of what she enjoyed—to golf or tend to her plants or play bridge or socialize. But since Brenda's attempted healing, Mom had not complained to me. I don't think she wanted to add any pressure to my health challenge.

As I got up to leave, I leaned over and kissed my mother's cheek. "Mom," I said, "you're so brave for forging on the way you do without complaining."

She said, "You're the one who's brave."

We choose some of our memories; others choose us. Mom became more reticent as time went on. Her comment that day was not the last thing she said to me in her difficult remaining months, but it was the nicest. It's the one I like to remember.

Elaine was a retired choir director and five-year ovarian cancer survivor. After she recovered, she recorded several favorite songs and sold the CDs to raise funds for cancer research. My friend Shelley bought a CD from her and asked her to deliver it to me in person. Elaine joined me for a cup of green tea at my kitchen table. We talked about our travails. She gave me fresh hope.

At my second to last chemo infusion, I listened to Elaine's CD. The intravenous steroids I received boosted my spirits. I felt relieved that surgery and radiation were behind me, glad that I had just one chemo to go, and elated that my treatment seemed to be working. The side effects from radiation had worn off. I could pee again without pain, a simple privilege I had not appreciated enough.

Elaine sang "Whistle a Happy Tune" and "Pennies from Heaven." I listened distractedly. I am astounded by songwriters like Cole Porter or the Gershwins. The ability to match the perfect lyric to a great tune knocks me out. But songs are personal, and those Elaine was singing weren't resonating. Then she broke into "On A Wonderful Day Like Today." My skin began to tingle. Despite the toxic chemicals now pumping into my bloodstream, I felt exhilarated. Elaine's delivery was upbeat. The lyrics, equally so. Knowing what my new friend had gone through, and how she had prevailed, made the song even more inspiring. I am one of those people who can't resist moving her head to the beat during a concert, not to mention lip-synching. I try to shake my head up and down instead of sideways to minimize the disturbance to anyone behind me. Now, lying in a hospital bed, I could not sit still.

Moving slowly so as not to disrupt the plastic tube connecting my chest to the drip bag, I swung my legs over the side of the bed and lowered my feet to the floor. Wheeling the I.V. bag rack beside me, I padded in my socks to the room entrance and closed the door. I lowered the blinds on the window overlooking the hall. No one who happened to walk by could see into the room as I picked up Chemo Bear, held him in my arms, and danced. Chemo Bear proved a perfect dance partner. He was soft and snugly and he followed my every step.

In the last verse, Elaine sings:
Let me take this occasion to say
That the whole human race should get down on its knees
Show that we're grateful for mornings like these
On a wonderful day like today.

Still holding Chemo Bear, I took Elaine's advice. I got down on my knees on the cool linoleum floor, and I bowed my head. I thanked God for bringing me this far. My heart filled with gratitude for competent medical treatment and caring doctors, for the knowledge of what I had been through and the prospect of finishing this ordeal before long.

In that brief, glorious song and steroid-inspired instant, I still did not see how meeting Elaine and hearing this song were part of a greater picture. But I did manage to banish from my head the possibility that all this treatment might not work. For that moment, I was convinced God wanted me well.

On Christmas Day up north, Burton and I babysat for Alexis while Andy and Amy went downhill skiing. I changed a diaper filled with contents the color of which was currently fashionable in interior design and thought back to the previous year. On that Christmas Day Andy and I had gone skiing together at Boyne Highlands in northern Michigan. One advantage of being Jewish is getting to ski on Christmas Day. The slopes are quiet. Few snowboarders come barreling toward you from above, snow grinding beneath their edges. There are no lines waiting for the chairlift. Andy and I skied the same runs that day—Heather, a gradual intermediate slope (my favorite) and Challenger, steeper and more advanced, the one Andy preferred. He skied faster than I did and waited for me at the bottom to ascend the chairlift together. After lunch, we took a few extra runs, making the most of a cold but sunny day. I loved having Andy all to myself, a rare privilege since he got married.

My mind skipped further back, to Christmas Day two years before, also at Boyne Highlands. I had gone skiing by myself. Twice in the past, I tore a knee ligament from falling on a ski slope, so I generally ski with caution. Feeling bold that afternoon, I stayed on Challenger. It featured a generous stretch of rare, winter sunlight and a chair-lift operator who greeted me like a long-lost good buddy each time I reappeared.

I spent that afternoon thinking about several friends. They were bright and vital, and they died too young. I decided I owed it to them to make the most of the day. I dedicated one ski run to Tavy, a brilliant fashion editor of the *Detroit News*. (Tavy wrote hundreds of creative columns. My favorite was one she penned on a 1970s skimpy, fashion fad called "hot pants" which she deemed inappropriate for women of a certain age. It concluded with a poem. I still remember the last lines. "Unless your legs are perfect joys/Short little shorts are for short little boys.") I dedicated one run to Marji, an equally talented fashion editor of the *Detroit Free Press* who once, when doing a feature on high-heeled pumps, photographed them on a gasoline pump.

Marji had recommended me for my first job in Detroit. And one to Jackie, the savvy owner of the cutting-edge gallery where I bought several artworks by Detroit artists. At the end of her life, Jackie had insisted on attending my fiftieth birthday party, the last social engagement she was able to make. Tavy, Marji and Jackie, and too many other friends, had died of cancer.

Thankfully unaware of what lay beyond that ski slope for me, I made several runs that afternoon. Now I wondered how I had ever had such stamina. When Alexis laid down for a nap, so did I.

Back in Detroit, five days later I underwent what I prayed was my last round of chemo ever. My final, finito, forever last round. On our way out of the chemo ward, Burton held the door for me. Stepping through, I thrust my arms overhead and whooped.

Burton gave me a hug. "You did it," he said in a husky voice.

"We did it," I said. We high-fived. And high-tenned.

The mix of emotions we felt reminded me of the time we drove a rented van with our young sons up north in winter. Just after we passed Chuck's Corner, we hit a patch of black ice, and the vehicle skidded and spun. Dark fir trees flashed in front of us, then field, then fir, then field, then fir. The vehicle leaned from one side to the other, threatening to overturn, but righted itself at the last minute. Burton slowed to a stop and we waited for our heartbeats to return to normal. Now, too, we felt relieved but shaky. Over the past five months, I had survived countless spinouts of fear, along with major surgery, radiation and chemo. Burton had been with me every mile of the way. My thyroid problem still loomed, but for that moment I managed to put it out of my head. Burton and I reveled in how far we had come.

The next afternoon, my sister called. "You were my hero of the year," she said.

"Next year I hope someone else wins that title."

That night, New Years Eve of 2004, we attended a dinner party at Barbara and Freddy's house. When we toasted to good health, all the guests at the long rectangular table nodded at me. Zina and Michael, who had visited and called so often over the past few months, carried their flutes over to clink with mine. Several guests were just casual acquaintances, but they all were aware of my plight. When cancer hits, word spreads fast. Even in the middle of an elegant dinner party, everyone knows how vulnerable they are. Cancer can strike whenever and whomever it chooses. It is an equal-opportunity attacker. One person's battle is everyone's battle.

Just before we returned to Florida, we visited Dr. Malone. Again, the sign outside the small examining room read Farbman/Malone. The little plaque advising patients to have hope remained propped in a corner. I remembered how dazed and fearful I was the first time I met my oncologist. I had come to cherish him. I appreciated his dry sense of humor and his willingness to take or promptly return my anxious phone calls, his ability to settle me down with a smart and matter-of-fact response. I was grateful for his surgical expertise, grateful that the less-drastic hysterectomy he had performed allowed me to again pee and poop without problems.

Dr. Malone leafed through the paperwork on my recent tests. He patted the sheaf of papers and smiled. "As good as we could have hoped," he said. "I consider you cured … until proven otherwise."

"All right!" I exclaimed. I jumped up and, for the first time, I hugged him. I stepped back and looked into his caring blue eyes. "Thank you. For everything."

He hugged me back, awkwardly, with one arm. Dr. Malone wasn't a touchy-feely sort. His ruddy cheeks turned a deeper shade of pink.

My chemo port still bulged out on my chest. The skin over it remained stretched and sore.

"Can we take out my port?" I asked.

He shook his head. "Let's leave it in for a while. Just in case."

We returned to Longboat Key, to the same rental house we had occupied a year ago, the house in which I had woken ten months before with a sudden pain my groin. We were overjoyed to look out the window again at the sparkling aquamarine Gulf of Mexico.

Burton stood next to me at the salt-laced window watching for the graceful arching of dolphins in the blue sea. "There were times I wondered if we'd ever get back," he said.

The first day we walked the beach, I tired quickly and needed to turn back in ten minutes. Four days later, using a cart, I played nine holes of golf. My swing had abandoned me. My shots skittered along the fairway. But at least I was playing, and it no longer hurt to swing through.

We spent three weeks in which I didn't see a doctor or feel the sting of a needle, smell anything antiseptic or worry about my latest test result. Each day, as my last round of chemo wore off, I walked a little farther on the beach or played an extra hole of golf. I relished the chance to take charge of my body and my schedule again and willed myself not to think of what still lay ahead.

I felt giddy from my new freedom and ready to spend money on myself—something I hadn't done in months. I hate to waste. I'll keep leftover roast chicken for days in case I might want it for lunch. Burton, who doesn't appreciate leftovers, often conducts search-and-destroy missions through the refrigerator. Suddenly, just as I happen to be home for lunch and have a yen for roast chicken, there is available glass shelf space where, the day before, I had to stack the Greek yogurt on top of the can of mixed nuts. The roast chicken upon which I had balanced the week-old loaf of rustic bread has disappeared along with the bread, and I have to content myself with cheese scrambled eggs. As part of my parsimony, I'm thrilled to find bargains. I brag about them when I do. Some of my cutest t-shirts are from Target. I combine errands to the post office, the bank and the market so as not to waste gas and did so before the term "ecology" entered American consciousness. Other than my exorbitant wig, since the previous July I hadn't bought a thing for myself. Why buy a new skirt or sweater if I wouldn't feel well enough (live long enough?) to wear it?

We drove past a wig shop. "Let's stop," I said.

Burton pulled the car into a parking space. "This isn't my thing," he said. "I'll wait here."

Gertrude, I had discovered, had issues. She needed constant tending. Fresh from the salon, she was on her best behavior. She looked shiny and fluffy for a day or two, but soon she started to droop and need professional service again. I could not shampoo or style her as I could if she were my own hair.

A friend told me about a friend of hers—a chemo patient who bought several synthetic wigs in different styles and colors. She washed them in the sink at night and popped them back on in the morning. She could be a new person from one day to the next. I wish I had thought of that, I said.

I admire women with the courage to display their bald heads during chemo or after. I wasn't that brave, and my bare skull felt cold. Tiny dark shoots had begun to sprout aloft, but it would be several weeks before I sported enough growth to term it hair or to venture out without covering my head.

The wig shop was a wonderment of styles and colors. Dozens of synthetic wigs sat on Styrofoam forms perched on shelves. I tried on flips and long, wavy numbers. I tried on blondes and blacks. I tried on one that was short and coppery, cropped in the feathery shag Meg Ryan made famous in the mid-1990s movie *French Kiss*. At the time, I had tried to copy the style but lacked sufficient follicles to create the desired textural effect. I looked more drowned rat than French flair.

The name of the wig was Frenchie. It cost $100.

"Frenchie it is," I said to my saleswoman. "I feel like being a redhead."

Our three weeks of freedom skidded to a halt. It was time to return to Detroit to face the tumor in my thyroid. My mood plummeted. The day before we were scheduled to fly home, we took a walk on the beach. It was then that I spied four women enjoying drinks on a blanket in the sand and felt drawn to them. I didn't realize it until the words came out of my mouth, but I wanted to give them a message. To impress upon them how lucky they were, how fleeting life, and health, can be. Why I thought they needed to hear such wisdom from me, I'll never know.

My approaching these strangers in the first place was out of character. They were clearly having a good time without me. While I appear to be outgoing, it's a front. I hide my self-consciousness the best I can, even from myself. I remember the very night I taught myself to engage socially. It was in 1977, the day Jimmy Carter became president. My brother-in-law Bob, Anne's late husband, served as one of Carter's campaign aides. He invited Burton and me to an inaugural gala at the Corcoran Gallery in Washington, D.C. Even though I had supported Michigander Gerald Ford's bid for a second term, I could not resist a chance to hobnob with political big shots and to admire fine art in the process. I expected to be part of an elite group of a few hundred. In fact, thousands of guests squeezed into a large two-level space, all looking to see who they knew or wanted to know. The only one I recognized was Congresswoman Bella Abzug, identifiable in one of her trademark hats, and surrounded by dozens of people. After a couple of nerve-enhancing drinks, I decided to conduct an experiment. I theorized that if I acted like someone people should know, they would think I was. I glided around making eye contact, extending my hand, saying, "Glad you could come!" or "Great to see you!" or "How've you been?" I approached more than fifty individuals or couples this way. Every single one returned my greeting warmly. Not one asked if or how they knew me. The experience taught me to handle a cocktail party the way Nijinsky handled a stage.

But early social insecurities stick with us. Underneath I'm still the awkward seventh-grader who entered a private girls' school knowing only one friend, my across-the-street neighbor Bobbye who had started in an earlier grade and was already popular, plus skilled at field hockey and tennis, other social assets I lacked. Throughout my six years at Kingswood, I often felt excluded by classmates I would have called "cool"—girls whose fathers tended to be auto execs for the then-Big Four, who lived in rambling farm colonial or Tudor homes in Bloomfield Hills, who owned multiple Fair Isle sweaters and new Weejun penny loafers and had lots of boyfriends from Cranbrook, the boys' school. None of those qualifications applied to me. My father was a blueprinter; I lived in a smaller home in Huntington Woods, several miles from tony Bloomfield Hills. I had two Fair Isle sweaters, a pair of worn Weejuns, and a relative dearth of Cranbrook admirers. The latter defect, I prefer to think, resulted from my being stingier with the family jewels than some other more generous and better-endowed classmates. My desire to be included may also stem from having been dropped in sorority rush from final desserts (the last stage before being invited to join) by AEPhi at the University of Michigan. Although I preferred and joined SDT, I still wanted to be asked. I even feel happy at the supermarket when I swipe my credit card, and the little screen sanctions me: Approved.

Despite my acquired social skills, approaching several strangers on a beach was out of character. I must have felt they'd want to meet me. That I had something so valuable to say that it was worth interrupting their revelry, risking their rejection. I don't know where I found the nerve to march up to them, especially with my husband trying to discourage me. Now I think it was because I was meant to meet them. I hope that every year they continue getting together. And that whenever they sip cocktails on that beach, their past encounter with the pale stranger in the grey chemo cap makes them enjoy their time together even more. Probably they don't remember me. But maybe they do. Maybe they even lift a glass of champagne to me. The cosmos works that way. We don't necessarily know the effect we have on others. I know I've never forgotten that meeting, or the woman in the navy blue sweatshirt who stood up and gave me a hug, or how hopeful she made me feel.

Later that day in Florida, I received still more signs. In a drafty Chinese restaurant I heard about a cancer survivor from my hometown who had two sons and who spelled her name the same way I did. Soon after, in a theater, mythical gods encouraged me to keep moving forward. If any one of those events had happened by itself, I would have deemed it a blessing and moved on. But one, two, three. A hat trick of surprises. Something significant was happening. Something that deserved my attention.

Riding home from the theater that night, I felt giddy. I had the same heart-expanding sense of possibility I'd felt on my first date with Burton when he slung his arm across the back of my chair at *Dr. Zhivago* and his hand alighted on my shoulder and stayed there.

"Godsigns," I said. "The things that happened today. Crazy as it sounds, I think they're signs from God."

If Burton hadn't been paying attention, or if he had pooh-poohed the notion or told me to screw my head back on and make sure my face pointed forward, I might have let the idea go. The truth is, Burton was so focused on making me well and doing what he could to cheer me up that he would probably have supported any oddball notion I came up with short of driving off the bridge for the thrill of it.

"I like the way you're thinking," he said. It was the punch line of a joke I've since forgotten. But it was what I needed to hear.

"Some amazing things happened today," I said. "Actually, they've been happening since I got sick. I saw them as individual events. Now I'm not so sure. One blessing, then another and another, back to back."

"Like winning the triple crown," Burton said. Burton loves anything to do with horses.

"Up to now, I've been so focused on trying to look forward that I forgot to look back. I didn't connect the dots. I didn't see the bigger picture."

Thinking about some of the events that had occurred in recent weeks, I ticked them off with my fingers. "The message

I picked in Ginger's labyrinth, 'Ask and Ye Shall Receive.' The hymn Eric sang. 'Footprints in the Sand.' Brenda's angel cards."

"Running into Larry at Duggan's after thirty-some years and hearing his cancer-survival story."

"Exactly."

"Why do you think they happened?"

"Because I needed them."

"Because you were looking for them?"

"Maybe. Does it matter?"

Burton drew his hand through his silver hair. Having recently turned sixty-two, he still had lovely, soft hair. "I guess not."

"What matters is they happened. And they gave me hope."

"Some people would call them coincidences."

Our tires hummed as we drove across the drawbridge at New Pass, over the channel that connects the Gulf with the bay and Lido Key with Longboat Key. We had never owned a boat in Sarasota. But when friends invited us on theirs, I jumped at the chance. I especially loved viewing the stately homes overlooking this stretch of water.

"Coincidences with a special purpose," I said, quoting Naven R. Johnson, a quirky character played by Steve Martin in his comedy, *The Jerk*. Naven has sex for the first time and writes home to his black sharecropper family that he has at last discovered his "special purpose." Burton and I saw the movie in 1979 when it came out and had watched it several times since. *The Jerk* remained one of our favorites.

"In AA, coincidences are called 'God's way of staying anonymous,'" I said. "Deepak Chopra thinks we increase the chance of coincidences by being open to them. I want to be open to them. To believe in them. Does that sound crazy?"

"If it helps, go for it."

"I want to see them as signs from God. Godsigns."

Burton, who had been with me through every scan, every needle, every knife, every anxiety pang, stopped for the traffic light by Publix. He turned to me and put his hand on mine.

"Godsigns," he said. "Why not?"

Early in the twentieth century, Swiss psychiatrist Carl Jung gave a name to the sort of coincidences that had been occurring since I was diagnosed. He deemed them synchronicity. According to Jung, for an event to represent synchronicity, certain characteristics apply. It is meaningful to the person perceiving it. It contains an emotional charge. There is psychic tension occurring in the perceiver—he or she is working on or worried about something. It has special timing, as in the Greek concept of *kairos*, that things come into our lives at important moments. It is outside of ego control. And it fits into some larger narrative or pattern in our life, which we may or may not yet understand.

All of those characteristics applied to the experiences I saw that night as Godsigns. The larger pattern came to me later. It was a tendency I had fought for much of my life. Despite Jane Fonda's claim that we mellow in our third acts, my sense of personal insecurity had grown. I once heard a profound Chinese saying: As we grow older, we become more of who we are. I wish I had become more secure as I grew older. But marriage troubles, increasing age (and its loyal advance team of sags, spots and memory lapses), and now a life-threatening disease had further taxed my self-confidence. My sense of personal insecurity might have stemmed from friction between my parents as I was growing up. It might have been something I inherited or learned from my mother or father. (Both seemed to feel that they didn't live up to their ancestors' reputations. Mom's mother was a beauty and a socialite; her father, a successful realtor. Dad's mother had started and grown the blueprint company Dad struggled to keep afloat; her brothers included a world-renowned architect, an engineer who designed the Hoover Dam and a steel magnate.) My insecurity might have resulted from a trans-generational wounding common among Jewish people after centuries of persecution. Our brains contain hundreds of millions of neurons firing hundreds of times a minute. So many experiences go into building our brains and making us who we are.

Whatever the reasons, rather than relax into life, I lived on guard, fearing the worst. I wanted to let my anxiousness go. I longed to overcome my habit of viewing worry as some sort of disaster insurance, as though anticipating the worst could somehow prevent it from sneaking up on me. Pow. Right in the kisser.

I yearned to sway with the wind like the willow tree in front of our farmhouse. I wanted to think more like author Byron Katie, one of my self-help gurus. She embraced whatever happened to her, even a painful cornea disease called Fuchs' dystrophy, a name I can't forget as Fuchs (rhymes with cukes) was my maiden name. Growing up in the sexually-repressed 1950s with a name that demanded precise penmanship and pronunciation, I quaked through every new roll call. Katie claims to have let go of reactionary fears, of what she calls her "story," and to have replaced them with optimism and joy.

It should be a simple goal to substitute loving thoughts for fearful ones. As the *Course in Miracles* says, pure love cancels out fear. But our egos, those champions of fear, are relentless. We may think we've suppressed them, but they rear up at any chance they get. Fear is their M.O. Turning around my thinking was as big a challenge as ridding my body of cancer, only no radiation machine has yet been developed to eradicate bad thoughts. I hoped Godsigns could be an antidote, a reminder to smile, to let go and to trust.

I longed to become more carefree. Not so carefree that I'd show up in a red hat and a purple dress, though Jenny Joseph makes a good case for them in her insightful poem, "Warning." It begins: *"When I am an old woman I shall wear purple / With a red hat which doesn't go and doesn't suit me."* The poem inspired the creation of the Red Hat Society. As much fun as the red-hatted ladies seemed to be having when I ran across them in restaurants, I was too style-conscious to indulge in such a fashion folly. Unless Vera Wang happened to show red and purple, that is, and I could pick up a bargain at Kohl's. But, a little more carefree wouldn't hurt. Maybe just enough to spring for the hat.

The word coincidence comes from Latin. From the words *cum*, meaning with or together, and *incidere*, to happen. Scientific theory contends that coincidence does not prove a causal relationship. If something is not replicable, hence provable, it is not deemed scientific. In considering recent coincidences, I chose to overlook scientific rationality. To see matters my way, the On High way.

Jung believed individuals could have "numinous" or awe-inspired experiences. My back-to-back experiences that day in Florida came wrapped in gossamer tissue with a big, gold bow on top. They were better than any Christmas morning, even when I did believe in Santa Claus. They filled me with awe and gratitude. Rational or not, I saw them as the universe's way of helping me to lighten up, to don a red hat in my heart, if not on my head.

Jung saw the Self as a force for organization. Words are one of the ways we organize. I have always loved words. I love to know them and to learn them and to shoot them around in my head as though they were cat's eye marbles. I love to use them, like Fancy Nancy of the children's books, who constantly drops fancy words and identifies them as such. I like puns, even when they make people groan. I enjoy making words up. That night in the car on the way home from the theater was the first time I organized a number of inspiring experiences into a pattern. The first time I gave them a name. To name something is to claim it. A baby, a friend, an idea—to name it is to nurture it.

Once I named these coincidences, I began to look for, and to find, others. Some would be even more improbable than those I had already experienced. I came to believe that God speaks in many ways and appears in many forms. Especially when we pay attention, when we need Him most. We pay attention best when we're vulnerable—that's a fancy word for hurting. When we're not so busy attending meetings and answering emails and making dates and thinking we're in charge. When we're not too busy to notice, God gives us signs.

Often these signs come from encounters with others. For me, that afternoon on the beach I had encountered an angel. Granted, she came with a navy blue sweatshirt and a glass of champagne, not the winged, haloed, gilded version depicted in art history. In the Bible, angels can appear in human form. When Joseph wanders the fields in search of his brothers, a stranger tells him where they moved their flock. Rabbis interpret this stranger to have been an angel. Without him, Joseph might never have found his brothers and been sold into slavery. He might never have risen to power in Egypt and, ultimately, saved the Hebrew nation. Angels in the Torah are considered *mal'akh Elohim*, messengers of God.

Some might consider me naïve and conclude that the universe has more important things to do than deal in hocus-pocus. Some deny the possibility of divine intervention altogether. Woody Allen says, "Not only is there no God, but try getting a plumber on weekends." Other nonbelievers demand an explanation for the Holocaust or suicide bombers. For Bernie Madoff's stealing the dreams of hard-working people. For earthquakes in Haiti. Oil spills in the Gulf. For deadly tornados and floods.

Smarter people than I don't know why bad things happen. I only know that good often comes out of bad. And that anyone enrolled in earth school long enough will face tough lessons. I also know the universe brings gifts as well as hardships. Whoever doesn't appreciate those gifts forfeits a chance for greater peace of mind.

I've come to believe in a God who speaks to each of us—rich or broke, thoughtful or selfish, healthy or sick. He speaks in English, Spanish, Swahili, Mandarin. He speaks in every language through our hearts. He speaks in clues, in riddles, in so-called chance encounters, in natural phenomena. Whether we ascribe to a religion or not, God gives us signs. We choose whether or not to see them.

I'd like to remain as certain of this all-knowing, all-giving, all-compassionate divine force as I was that night on our way home from the theater. I'd like to be more consistently joyful. There are times when my husband snaps at me, times when I worry about my children or grandchildren or witness an accident, and I feel less sanguine. When CNN interviews the parents of a soldier killed in the line of duty or I come across an article on the victims of sex offenders, I, too, wonder how a sympathetic, loving God can permit such heartache.

But Glory Hallelujah for the other days. Days when my hormones (what's left of them) cooperate or I watch a grandchild swim for the first time or score a rare birdie. Days when the sky is unbearably blue and I smell a sprig of fresh lavender, I am right there with Robert Browning. "... *the lark's on the wing; the snail's on the thorn; God's in His Heaven—All's right with the world!*"

Over the next weeks, despite my discovery of Godsigns, my faith would come and go. But that night in Florida, I believed. I believed God knew how much I dreaded heading home to face more tests, needles and knives, more worry and burned flesh. Through people on a beach and in a restaurant, through actors on a stage, He reassured me once again. I could, as they say in AA, "let go and let God." He was so on the case.

CHAPTER 13

Twinkle, Twinkle Little Star

*Those who are willing to be vulnerable
move among mysteries.*

—**Theodore Roethke**

CANCER TEACHES US to make the most of good days. Back in Detroit in late January, David asked me to shop for furniture with him. Other than for groceries, I hadn't shopped with either of my sons in many years. I learned my lesson on a visit to Hudson's at Northland Mall. Seeking to buy a top for myself, I was checking out a rack of blouses. Within seconds, I realized I had lost track of my little boys. It didn't take long to figure out where they were. A nearby rack of skirts began to sway violently, followed by grunts and shrieks and name-calling.

More than twenty years later, despite the winter gloom and snow, I relished the chance to spend time with my now much better behaved older son. A shopping excursion with him would provide fine bonding time. And focusing on a project always helped me to forget my troubles.

As a design editor, I knew the importance of scale. One of the biggest mistakes a homeowner can make is to purchase furniture without first checking room measurements. I stopped at David's ranch house with my metal tape. David held one end; I, the other, and we measured the living room. I made a rough sketch showing the overall size of the room and the locations of the fireplace, hearth and openings, and drew in an outline of the approximate best size of furnishings.

With the plan tucked in my purse, David and I started on Orchard Lake Road in West Bloomfield. At the first store, my son was not inspired. We left quickly. At the second, David spotted low, squarish, ochre-yellow leather side chairs.

"What do you think, Mom?"

I nodded. "The color will work with anything. They're masculine. Modern enough to be cool and big enough to hold two at a party. Good choice."

David handed over his credit card. I smiled, realizing I had never shopped with him before when he paid the bill.

We drove to Birmingham. At the Pita Café, we shared a plate of lamb shawarma with hummus. One advantage of living in an area with the largest population of Arabs outside the Middle East is great Lebanese food. Over dinner, David wondered if he should have negotiated a better price for the side chairs.

"The price was good already," I said.

"I should have tried," he said.

Across the street, we visited Arhaus. In the lower level, David admired a large, low, dark wood Asian-inspired coffee table with curved legs. I was pleased to see how sophisticated his taste had become.

We climbed the stairs. David found a salesperson.

"What discount can you give me?" he asked.

"Sorry. We don't discount," the man said. "We deliver for free."

"What about for cash?"

The man shook his head. "Sorry."

"Can I speak to the manager?"

"I am the manager."

I bit my lip to suppress a grin.

"What if I pick it up myself?"

"We pride ourselves on service. Delivery is part of our service."

The grin won out, and I turned my head away.

"What do you think, Mom?"

I compressed my lips and shrugged. "We'll keep looking if you want to."

"You win," David said to the manager and took out his wallet.

The rest of the week was less entertaining. I underwent another round of CT scans and met with Dr. John Jacobs, the chief of nose and throat surgery at Karmanos. He advised me to see Dr. Gregorian, "the best person in the city with a needle." Months before, she had biopsied my neck as well as my pelvis. Burton and I drove to yet another hospital where Dr. G. numbed my neck and probed it with a needle. The tumor seemed to have shrunk and hardened, probably from chemo, she said. For more than half an hour, she pushed and prodded with different needles, trying to penetrate the tumor and remove cancer cells. I lay still, unnerved, wondering when this ordeal would end. I felt no pain but a lot of pressure on my throat. I wished I had taken a Valium.

At our next appointment, Dr. Jacobs said the biopsy showed the tumor in my neck was not thyroid cancer, which would have been treatable by swallowing radioactive iodine pills.

"The tissue suggests endometrial cancer," he said.

Dr. Jacobs looked to be at least fifty. Someone with the hospital had told me his patients consider him "a god." I figured he must have plenty of experience with cases like mine.

"How many metastases have you seen from uterus to thyroid?" I asked.

"None."

Air escaped my chest.

"How many other metastases to the thyroid?"

"One. A man with lung cancer."

Of all thyroid cancers, only one or two percent have spread from other tumors, he said. He recommended removing the half of my thyroid which contained the tumor. He called the surgery "tricky." The tumor lay near one of four parathyroid glands, which control the body's calcium levels. He could not tell from the CT scan whether the tumor had grown outside my thyroid gland or was encapsulated. Nor did the scan reveal whether the tumor touched the laryngeal nerve, which controlled my vocal cord.

"What happens if you damage a vocal cord?"

"You have two of them," he said. "Many people have only one that works and don't even know it."

To check the function of my vocal cords, he asked me to open my mouth, stare at the ceiling, hold still and breathe out while he inserted a slender metal probe. This loathsome test made my eyes tear and caused me to gag. On the third try, threatened with the even more abhorrent prospect of a probe down my nose if the route through my mouth failed to work, I managed not to gag. Dr. Jacobs determined that both of my vocal cords functioned.

"How will we know if one is damaged in surgery?"

"You might be hoarse for a while. Soon you'll be able to speak just fine, but you won't be able to carry a tune."

I scheduled a date for surgery but worried about Dr. Jacobs' lack of experience with my type of cancer. Burton found a leading thyroid surgeon in New York City and set up a phone consultation. The doctor assured us he knew Dr. Jacobs, respected his ability, and agreed with his approach.

"But he has no experience with uterine cancer of the thyroid," I said.

"Neither does anyone else."

In early February, as the New England Patriots beat the Philadelphia Eagles, the kids' friends whooped and cheered and graciously ignored me. The calm I felt on our last night in Florida had evaporated. At Andy and Amy's Super Bowl party, I wept through several downs. Not that I cared who won or lost. I wept because I was giving my seven-month-old granddaughter her bottle and my throat surgery would take place the next day. I worried about what the surgeon might find and whether he could remove the entire tumor. I worried I might never be able to sing Alexis another lullaby and hit the right notes. Even though I didn't have a pretty voice like my sister, I enjoyed singing and could carry a tune. I worried that I wouldn't live long enough to take Alexis shopping for whatever became the future equivalent of low-rise skinny jeans. I worried I wouldn't live long enough for my granddaughter to feel the same love for me that I felt for my grandmother. And because when you are scheduled for cancer surgery, worry is what you do.

Alexis stared at me with dark blue eyes, understanding everything.

After surgery, I was too groggy to write in my journal. Andy took notes for me when Dr. Jacobs visited my hospital room. He had removed half of my thyroid and half of one parathyroid gland. He said that ninety percent of the tumor was located inside the gland; ten percent outside. He did not know if the laryngeal nerve had been damaged. Although he had worked closer to the nerve than he liked, the surgery "went fine." The next day, another doctor removed the drain tube in my throat and put in a stitch. I knew I was allergic to penicillin, but now Clindamycin caused me to develop hives. I switched to a different antibiotic.

Three days after my thyroid surgery, Burton and I visited Dr. Jacobs' office. He approved of my incision and stopped my antibiotics.

"The tumor came off smoothly, but it was less than one millimeter away from the nerve," Dr. Jacobs said. "That's not as thick as a piece of paper." He tore a piece of paper off a prescription pad. "About like this," he said, handing the slip to me. I held it up sideways. The edge was so thin I could barely see it. I returned it with a scowl.

"There's a reasonable chance we got it all, but I'm not comfortable with the margin. I recommend following up with radiation."

The tumor he removed was clear cell or poorly differentiated, Dr. Jacobs said. Undifferentiated cells are hard to identify. Although the cellular structure resembled that of the tumor in my uterus, he wasn't sure it came from my uterus. It might also represent a second primary. I should have been comforted to realize my tumor may not have spread through my bloodstream, which could then continue to affect other organs. But mostly I was freaked out that not just one but two totally separate parts of my body could have been so disruptive.

Dr. Jacobs said he would test my vocal cord again at our next appointment when my neck was less sore. I dreaded submitting to another probe.

"You told me if I lost a vocal cord, I couldn't keep a tune."

"Right," he said.

Scratchy, but on key, I started to sing "Twinkle, Twinkle Little Star."

After the first two lines, he said, "You proved your point."

Five weeks after I finished chemo, the skin over my port had grown increasingly tender and begun to disintegrate. A black rubber knob started to protrude from my chest. Dr. Malone decided it had to come out.

Because we were scheduled to fly to Florida the next morning, Chuck, a technician in Interventional Radiology, agreed to work late. I again felt grateful that we had chosen a hospital small enough that staff members would do special favors. At about 4 p.m., I lay down on Chuck's operating table. He numbed my chest and turned on an x-ray machine. I could see the five-inch tube which snaked between my ribs and connected the rubber-covered titanium head to a vein.

Receiving my port had been simple. A surgeon implanted it during my hysterectomy while I was sedated, Removing it proved grueling. The procedure took close to two hours as Chuck numbed the area, cut away dead skin and stitched up living skin. Instruments rested on the gown over my belly. I had to lie still. I felt pressure on my chest, smelled alcohol, heard the hiss of a blade.

"This blade is dull," Chuck said. "It worked fine this morning."

"Ha-ha," I said.

Sensing how nervous I was, Chuck kept the wisecracks coming.

I asked if he was using dissolving stitches.

"If they gave me what I asked for."

"Gallows humor," I said.

"I haven't drunk that since college."

In the background, music played. Bill Withers sang, "You can call on me, brother, when you need a hand. We all need someone to lean on." I thought about all the doctors and nurses and friends I had leaned on over the past few months. About my husband, the best person I knew in a crisis, who waited at that moment in a lobby for me. I thought about Chuck, with his corny jokes, and his nurses Kevin and Carlos, all of whom had stayed late to help me.

Kevin grabbed a tissue and dabbed at my eyes.

"Don't move," Chuck warned. "If you drop those instruments, I'll have to call the instrument police."

After, I wrote in my journal. *I haven't just been pulling rabbits out of hats, I've been pulling out great big, fluffy Easter bunnies. I hope my streak continues.*

Two pain-free/doctor-free weeks in Florida raced by. With stitches in my chest, I could not risk swinging a golf club. But we rode our bikes to Publix on Longboat Key. We walked the beach. We dined out with friends. The swelling in my neck diminished. Six stubborn, white tendrils, about one-half inch long, waved from my skull. I admired their endurance when their less hardy comrades had long since defected. The deserters now showed signs of reappearing, but the emerging stubble was so short it was velvety to the touch but barely visible. I pulled on Frenchie and kept going. For most of the time, I remembered my Godsigns and kept my fears in check. I almost felt like a healthy person again.

In late February, we flew back to Detroit and drove to the Weisberg Clinic to meet again with Dr. Forman. I trudged past Felicia at the reception desk, returning her So-glad-to-see-you! with a weak smile. Remembering how radiation had scorched my pelvis, I dreaded what it might do to my neck.

"There's a thirty to sixty percent chance some cancer was left in your throat," Dr. Forman said at my appointment. "I've talked to Drs. Malone and Jacobs. We all agree. There's a fifty percent chance the tumor will grow back. If we radiate, that chance drops to five percent."

Dr. Forman proposed 5,000 units of radiation, to be delivered over twenty-five days. Unlike the pelvis, where it was difficult to avoid affecting other healthy organs, the throat was relatively easy to radiate, he said. An intensity-modulation system allowed the beam to wrap around critical structures—the trachea, esophagus and pharynx. The recurrent laryngeal nerve should not be affected. Studies showed radiation to be most effective when given within six weeks of surgery.

I grimaced. What about side effects?

The treatment should have little impact on my ability to eat, speak or swallow, he said. The worst side effect: a temporary sore throat and redness of the skin on my neck.

"We want to do everything possible to eliminate all the cancer from your body," he said. And then he added the ultimate deal clincher. "Our goal is to cure you."

As I plodded back into the Weisberg Center, I thought: This cannot possibly be as bad as it sounds. I had returned to have a mask made of my face. The mask would be bolted to the radiation table to immobilize my head. Once this mask was made, I would be pinned beneath it for about half an hour, five days a week for five weeks. The mask would ensure that I lay still and that my neck received a precise beam. Misdirected radiation could otherwise damage my recurrent laryngeal nerve or my trachea, affecting my ability to speak, breathe or swallow.

Crowded elevators and tight spaces cause me to hyperventilate. Still, I lay down on the table and told myself, *You know how important this is. You can do it.*

"This will feel warm at first; it will cool off quickly," the technician said.

I watched her lower a full-face plastic mask, filled with soft, hot foam, toward me. The mask drew closer until warm foam pressed against my skin and the contraption was locked to the table. My vision blurred. The foam felt like suffocating slime. The air was thick and steamy. Unable to move my head, I tried to pray, to visualize a peaceful lake setting up north, to remember my Godsigns, to know this would end soon. But panic flooded through me. My heart raced. I gasped for air. My eyes teared over.

I banged on the table with my fists. Through clamped teeth, I yelled, "Get me out of here!"

A technician unlocked the mask. I wheezed gallons of air, then gulped from a glass of water. Over seven months I had lived through a hysterectomy, six rounds of chemo, thirty-three days of radiation, emergency surgery to remove my port, surgery to remove part of my thyroid and too many scans and needles to count. I had found my limit.

Dr. Forman came in.

"I'm sorry," I said, still gasping. Tears spilled down my cheeks. I was dooming my outcome. What a loser I was. "I can't do this."

He shook his head. "Truth is I couldn't either," he said. He turned to a technician. "Go to an alpha cradle."

Minutes later, my heart slowed to normal. I lay down again, the back of my head resting in a soft bed of warm foam. It cooled and hardened in the shape of my skull. The alpha cradle would not hold me as still as the mask which Dr. Forman preferred, but it was tolerable.

Soon after, at a funeral home, Ruth stood in front of me in line. We waited to express our condolences to the family of the deceased. I hadn't seen Ruth for several years. Her daughter had attended Cranbrook with my son Andy.

Ruth was a handwriting analyst who had once analyzed my penmanship. She told me the large size of my writing indicated a desire to be noticed; the verticality, that I was practical and independent. The ascending baseline, she said, meant that I was optimistic. Now I wished I were as optimistic as she thought.

"I remember you changed your handwriting," Ruth said.

"You're right," I said.

In my thirties, I gave up the right-slanting style of cursive I had been taught as a child. It looked awkward and immature, unlike the graceful script of my mother-in-law, who had been a schoolteacher and whose handwritten notes appeared so even and elegant. I switched to a rounder, vertical script.

"You became more authentic," Ruth said.

Ruth asked how I was. I told her about my treatment. I blurted out how I had failed to tolerate the mask. "It was worse than *Silence of the Lambs*. Hannibal Lecter wasn't pinned down."

Ruth told me her husband had gone through tonsil cancer. "He suffered through the mask and hated it. But his tonsil was removed." She put her hands on my shoulders and looked into my eyes. "And he's fine."

Ruth reached into her handbag, pulled out a slender silver chain, and told me to turn around. She fastened the chain around my neck. "Be strong," she said. "This is all the strength you'll need."

Ruth did not know how much I liked acorns. She had never visited my home in Franklin. She didn't know I had named it Acorn Hill and decorated it with acorn hardware and tiles.

Home later, I looked in the mirror and saw the charm that hung just below my collarbone. It could have been an angel or a heart or a flower or a star or any of thousands of charms sold in jewelry stores. It wasn't.

It was a delicate but unmistakable Godsign. A tiny silver acorn.

Cancer treatment is full of ups and downs. The night before my throat radiation began, Burton and I sat in our library. I wondered aloud how I could swallow without moving my head during radiation. I worried that my refusing the mask could compromise precision.

The phone rang. Dr. Forman.

"I spent a long time designing your radiation plan. The plan is good," he said. He factored in a five to seven millimeter variability, as opposed to the one millimeter allowance the mask would have permitted. "I'm confident I can treat the tumor while sparing critical structures."

A wave of hope spread through me.

"There's something else I need to tell you."

A tone in his voice turned my skin clammy.

"To create my radiation plan, I studied your latest CT scan. I observed a change in your neck. To be sure, I had two more radiologists examine the scan. We all agree. Something is growing there."

I was still sobbing when David called. "I'll be right over," he said.

Half an hour later, our older son walked in. He wore a black Nike warm-up suit. His face was still flushed from tennis. He sat on the sofa, wrapped his muscular arms around me, and started to cry.

"I took an extra twenty minutes so I wouldn't lose it like this," he said. "I'm not crying because I'm afraid anything bad is going to happen. I'm crying because you're my mom, and I love you so much."

That harmless-looking cone-shaped machine, those upbeat technicians had caused me such misery four months before. Back in the radiation room, I lay down again on the same cotton-sheet-covered, glass-topped table I had laid on half an hour a day for six and a half weeks the previous fall.

Instead of resting my legs in a plastic mold, I rested my head in the alpha cradle. Denise lined up the overhead machine with blue dots which were tattooed on my chest and skull at the time the cradle was made. To further help me hold still, she stretched a strip of masking tape across my chin and onto the table on either side. A warm, wet washcloth was draped across my neck. Denise called it a bolus, said it was meant to shorten the radiation beam. The approach seemed primitive, given the sophisticated technology that accompanied it. Denise left to operate the machine from the control room. The lead door clunked shut.

Five days a week, from twenty to thirty minutes a session, the machine moved and paused as it had before, this time shooting an invisible beam at points inside my neck. I refrained from swallowing while the machine whirred. I prayed. I gazed up at the backlit photograph still suspended overhead—Tahquamenon Falls in the Upper Peninsula. I thought about the visit Burton and I had made there a few years before. Burton's ADD had kicked in, and he'd grown restless spending so much time in Northern Lower Michigan. He decided that once a week we should go someplace new. I was content staying home and reading on my porch swing, but a happy husband mattered more. We played golf at different courses. We drove to the U.P. and saw the breathtaking Pictured Rocks on the southern shore of Lake Superior—pink, red and green sandstone bluffs that rise 200 feet from the water. We visited the Marquette Branch State Prison, a spooky Romanesque, stone building built in 1889 with arches and turrets and a gift shop selling items made by prisoners. Burton bought a carved wood back-scratcher with a red handle. It remains his favorite. He loses it periodically but eventually finds it again.

Burton was the restless one in our relationship, the one who said yes to chairing committees and events. Most often when Burton said yes, I grumbled at first but eventually pitched in and organized the trip or the dinner party or co-chaired the event.

Gazing up at rocks and waterfalls, I again felt the warmth of Burton's hand helping me climb over boulders and heard the sound of rushing water over the hum of the radiation machine. In spite of my initial resistance, I had to admit that Burton's restlessness had led to many fine adventures. I prayed there would be more.

CHAPTER **14**

I Hope You Dance

*Faith ... is about knowing, as Quakers would put it,
that there is an inextinguishable light inside everyone
that is holy. It's about valuing the holy in the face
of the flawed, about leaving room to grow, to fall
down, then get back up again, all with equal dignity.*

—Lise Funderburg, Looking Out For #2, *O, The Oprah Magazine*

WE WERE INVITED to Miami for a friend's seven-
tieth birthday party. When the invitation arrived, I declined.
I'd be undergoing radiation and expected I'd either feel too
depressed for such a gala occasion or would lack the strength.

Radiation to my neck proved less taxing than it did to my
pelvis, and my schedule gave us weekends off. Several days into
radiation, I still had energy. Cancer had not only taught me to
seize opportunities. It had deepened my already considerable
appreciation for friends. And I loved a good party. Especially
one that would take place at a glamorous palazzo once owned
by fashion designer Gianni Versace. Shelly and Joel were gracious and imaginative hosts. A few years before, Burton and I
had attended an unforgettable gala which Joel threw for Shelly's
fiftieth. Joel had secretly taken dance lessons and learned the
part of Erik, the phantom in *Phantom of the Opera*, when he
dances with Christine. Wearing a mask and accompanied by a

professional dancer, Joel surprised Shelly and all of us by performing at the soirée.

I called. Could we still come? Absolutely, Shelly said. And so we flew to Miami.

The scar from my recent surgery glared from the base of my neck, and the skin around it had begun to redden. But my old turquoise silk paisley Blumarine skirt fit and Gertrude was newly styled. Both, I decided, detracted from my irritated throat.

It was a balmy tropical night. Dinner was served under the stars in the walled courtyard of Casa Casuarina, a space surrounded by arched windows and adorned with columns and carved urns and tall palm trees. Guests danced on a clear plastic floor installed above a mosaic-tiled pool. On a balcony, a Latin singer with long, curly dark hair and a black fedora undulated her arms and hips. The beat and the music were irresistible. I was grateful to dance in such a magical setting and to wear bronze Manolo Blahnik sandals which proved comfortable and which I'd bought on sale. I was grateful to dance with a man who, despite some earlier lapses, had lately shown more love and support than I'd ever known. I was grateful that my pelvis had recovered enough to move my legs without pain.

At the end of one dance, a pretty blonde came up to me. Suzanne reminded me that we had met several years before when I'd scouted her house for a possible design feature. She had heard I'd been sick.

"How's it going?" she asked.

"So far, so good." I tapped my knuckles on my unusually fluffy head.

"Since I last saw you, I went through tongue cancer," she said.

I widened my eyes. "How are you?"

"I have some problems with my teeth. I don't salivate the way I used to. But it's been five years, and I'm here tonight."

"And you look great. What was your treatment?"

"Surgery. And so much radiation that for a while my lower face turned black."

I studied her. Big blue eyes. Classic profile. A fine scar on her neck—nothing I'd have noticed without looking for it. And no trace of a burn.

"Who treated you?"

"Dr. Jacobs and Dr. Forman."

My doctors.

I was so glad we had come.

We returned to Detroit. My spirits, and my faith, slumped again. The weather was cold and grey. I worried about what radiation was doing, and not doing, to my throat. My neck grew redder every day.

I had one fine distraction. When Barbara advised me to make plans, I took her advice. Burton and I had purchased a winter home in Laurel Oak, a golf community in Sarasota. The back of the house faced west, capturing the sunsets we enjoyed in our rental on the Gulf. The layout featured a master bedroom on one side of the house and guest bedrooms on the other. I was excited about the residence, but worried, too. I wondered how long we might enjoy our new home together.

Working on furnishings, I was driving on Maple Road to the Michigan Design Center in Troy to meet with Rick. He had helped me design our Franklin home and, as a favor, had rein-stalled my mom's old apartment in her new one. I punched my sister's number on my cell phone and turned on the speaker.

"You caught me on a ski slope," Anne said, her voice rising with enthusiasm. "I'm gazing at snow-covered mountains. Pine trees. Blue sky."

"Great," I said, trying to dredge up some happiness for her.

Anne deserved some fun. She had come through five rough years nursing her husband to an early death from a rare neu-roendocrine cancer. Now she had a fiancé with whom she was visiting Beaver Creek. I knew she meant to cheer me, but her gusto made me feel even sorrier for myself. I hung up as soon as I could.

I loved skiing so much that even when my contemporaries gave it up and I couldn't find anyone to join me, I still jumped in a car at Christmastime and drove an hour to ski by myself on molehills in northern Michigan. Now my sister, who never cared about the sport, was enjoying sunshine and groomed snow and thousands of feet of vertical drop while I might never have another chance to ski. God willing, cancer had been permanently eradicated from my pelvic bone and muscles, and I would be able to cruise down a mountain, even a hillside, again. Meanwhile I was stuck in Detroit, wondering when the cumulative effects of radiation would cause me a sore throat and problems swallowing. The temperature had dropped below thirty degrees; the road was slippery; and I was late for my meeting. If Rick billed me for the time I missed, I'd be aggravated. If he didn't, I'd feel guilty. I couldn't speed up because I was caught behind an old Ameritech pick-up truck. The other lane was blocked for road construction.

The light turned red, and the Ameritech repair truck pulled to a stop in downtown Birmingham near the old Jacobson's store, now an ad agency. (The Michigan-based luxury regional department store chain closed in 2002. As a young woman, I loved shopping at their Birmingham store where sales help treated you like family.) I drew to a stop behind the truck. Chafing that I wasn't the sister skiing out West, I glared at the truck's rusted rear fender. I scowled at the stuff strewn in the open bed—orange and white emergency cones, yellow temporary barricades, ropes, a ladder. What a mess. I sighed. Now I'd be even later.

Then I spotted it. And I shivered. I had been too busy feeling sorry for myself to notice. In the movie *Bruce Almighty*, God (Morgan Freeman) deputizes Bruce (Jim Carrey) to represent Him. Bruce tries to win back his girlfriend, Grace, (Jennifer Aniston) with special effects like heart-shaped clouds and bird formations spelling out: C A L L B R U C E.

That morning, I received divine reassurance from a rusty old Ameritech truck. The license plate was plain royal blue trimmed with white, not decked out with the Mackinac Bridge or a sunset over Lake Michigan or any other new design intended to make money for the Department of Motor Vehicles. This simple, no-fangled license plate was probably as old as the vehicle itself. No doubt the upper-right corner contained several layers of stickers indicating each year the license was renewed. The plate was dinged and bruised, the only one of its kind in the world, and it sat right in front of me. It took snow, road construction and a red light to force me to pay attention. My jaw fell open. My eyes widened. When the light changed, the driver behind me tooted, reminding me to accelerate.

My lucky number is 8; Burton's is 5. The number of that license plate: 8585MD.

For days I marveled at the message on that license plate. It was pure synchronicity. A sign of hope. A clear and amazing Godsign. Godsigns, I've come to believe, are like radio waves. They are constantly in the atmosphere, but we pick up on them best when we need them. When our emotional radio is tuned in. When we are alert and open to guidance.

Other survivors recount miracles of their own. Harvey, the psychiatrist I spoke to who'd had lung cancer, told me about something that happened just before he was diagnosed. "A client I hadn't seen for ten years called. She said she'd never had a dream in her life, but the night before, she had one. A man appeared to her and said, 'Tell Harvey to go to the doctor.'"

Geralyn Lucas relates a story in *Why I Wore Lipstick to My Mastectomy*. The day before her surgery, she rode in a cab. The driver, accelerating and braking to the tune of "La Bamba," told her she looked "hot." He wouldn't think so the next day, she lamented, after she lost her boob. The driver whipped the cab into a no-parking zone, jumped into the back seat, and took her hand. He promised her she'd be fine. He had survived testicular cancer. He said, "I have one ball."

Following a devastating stroke of her left hemisphere, brain scientist Jill Bolte Taylor moved home to Indiana to recover. In

My Stroke of Insight, she writes that she knew coming home was the right decision when the phone number she received turned out to be the exact date of her birth—day, month and year.

Godsigns are symbols. Jung believed a symbol could be true inside and false outside. He theorized that the significance of a symbolic event exists not in what happens but in how we feel about what happens. In what it represents to us. In the meaning we bring.

Psychoanalyst Elizabeth Mayer had an experience that sent her on a quest to discover the science behind what she terms "anomalous phenomena." Her daughter's treasured harp was stolen. After she failed for two months to locate the instrument through conventional means, a friend suggested she call a dowser. Doubtful but desperate, she phoned the president of the American Society of Dowsers, who proceeded to locate the instrument. As Dr. Mayer drove home from picking up the missing harp, she thought: This changes everything.

Extraordinary Knowing details Mayer's attempt to understand ESP, mental telepathy and other psychic phenomena. She writes, "To see a view of the world in which anomalous experience happens, we need to temporarily abandon a view of the world in which rational thought happens."

Rabbinic scholars interpret and reinterpret the Torah. In rethinking the story of Moses and the burning bush, rabbis sometimes turn it around. God did not simply burn within a single bush on the occasion that Moses spotted it. Rather, some sages say, countless bushes burned with the Creator's fire. The day that Moses saw one was the day he had eyes to see it.

Although quilting may date back as far as ancient Egypt, it was a popular American craft by the late eighteenth century. Handmade quilts consisted of symmetrical, geometric designs. In the late nineteenth century, a more spontaneous, free-form style developed. At the Philadelphia Centennial Exposition of 1876, the popular Japanese pavilion featured crazed ceramics and asymmetrical art. It opened the eyes of Victorian women to more expressive possibilities. It inspired a needlework trend called "crazy quilting." Victorian women began combining mis-matched pieces of velvet and silk and other exotic fabrics in random patterns, seamed with unusual stitching.

In the twenty-first century, with the Internet at our fingertips and spiritual traditions taking multiple forms, we are offered an array of possibilities. We can take as many pieces as we like, create our own crazy quilt of beliefs. I stitched together Godsigns from other-worldly phenomena like Brenda's angel cards and Marianne Williamson's *Course in Miracles* guidance. I stitched in advice from rabbis, from *Kabbalah* and Buddhism, from energy healers, from a Native American medicine wheel. I also stitched in Godsigns from more worldly experiences—encounters with strangers, conversations with friends. From numbers and from books. A crazy quilt of associations that work for me.

When we allow ourselves to see on an emotional level, we look beyond an event to the significance of the event. We find what matters to us. We create our own crazy quilt of wisdom, inspiration and insight. Godsigns need no explanation. They may not mean a thing to anyone else. To one who needs them, they are miracles, big and small. They wait for us to discover them, to derive their meaning, to catch our breath with wonder. To embrace them.

Godsigns nudge us into the light of hope and possibility. They are tiny oars that propel our life rafts through a sea of fears. They are the drink of water given to a runner on the verge of collapse, the second wind that spurs a biker on. They are manna from the universe that nourishes our hearts and our souls, that helps us to survive.

Godsigns come in many forms. Like Moses, we simply need eyes to see them.

As radiation wore on, the skin on my neck turned more tender. It changed from shell pink to radish red. My voice grew so hoarse that I sounded like a smoker with laryngitis. For the first four weeks, the radiation machine zapped eight areas, including a vocal cord. After a month, as swallowing solid foods began to feel like choking down large pills, the radiation field was narrowed. With my vocal cord no longer bombarded, my swallowing problems disappeared. My voice would take several months to return to normal. I cleared my throat before answering the phone.

Burton and I met with Dr. Forman every week. In one of our last appointments, he advised that tumor masses shrink slowly, that mine could continue to shrink for three months after radiation.

He added, "Your neck will continue to redden for a week or two."

That proved an understatement.

Like others I've met in the cancer field, Dr. Forman had a good heart, a great mind and a caustic wit. In a meeting near the end of my treatment, I noticed my file. It was over an inch deep

"That is a thick file," I said.

"Thick is good. People who die fast have thin files."

The annual Karmanos fundraising ball, for which Burton and I had accepted the honorary chairmanship, was six weeks away. I was scheduled for CT scans just before the event.

I said to Dr. Forman, "If I get bad results, I'll be a wreck."

"There's no reason to expect a bad report. If you got one, it would be more dramatic."

I said, "That logic stinks."

I endured radiation to my throat for five and a half weeks. On the last day, the machine finished its circuit around me and returned to a stop. It rested near tranquil Tahquamenon Falls, waiting for its next victim, appearing quiet and harmless once more.

Denise, in the control room, spoke over the intercom. "All done," she said.

"Yippee!" I shouted.

I tore the sheet from my body and flung it to the floor. I tossed the washcloth from my neck and kicked my feet and punched my hands in the air. Burton, who had witnessed my jubilation on the monitor, walked in along with Denise. They each wore matching grins. Denise pulled the tape from my chin and lowered the glass and steel radiation table.

I jumped down and pulled Denise to me and danced her around in circles. As we danced, I belted out, "goodbye, farewell, *auf Wiedersehen, adieu!*" Denise laughed and pumped my hand and joined me in singing.

Lee Ann Womack sings another song that causes me to tear up every time I hear it. It is about a mother's advice to her daughter, advice I hoped to pass on to any grandchildren I would be lucky enough to have. "When you get the chance to sit it out or dance/I hope you dance." I doubt Lee Ann had a radiation room in mind when she sang those lyrics. I bet the songwriters (Tia Sillers and Mark Sanders, whose identity I Googled) didn't either. But I was sure they'd approve.

As Dr. Forman predicted, the results of radiation continued to intensify after the treatment stopped. Each day for several weeks the skin on my neck became redder and rawer, a burned condition called radiodermatitis. My throat itched and stung and bled and crusted over with scabs. I slathered on salve which congealed in oozing, white patches.

Cancer treatments, and their side effects, have no regard for your social schedule. In April, Burton and I were invited to a wedding. As the date drew near, I had another appointment with Rick.

I wailed, "How can I show up at a wedding with my neck looking like this?"

"Suzy," Rick said in the same nonjudgmental voice he once used to convince me that a room should have a single focal point, "the point is you're *at* the party."

Whenever you feel sorry for yourself, count on the universe to remind you to buck up; there are worse problems.

The mother of the groom had lost her daughter, husband, father, best girlfriend and sister. Rather than destroy her, those deaths had left Jennifer determined to enjoy every minute. I hoped my flaming neck would not upset any of the guests at her son's upcoming wedding. Though I knew how she would feel, I warned her anyway.

"I look scary."

Jennifer said, "When you love someone, you don't care how they look. You just want them with you."

By some trick of fate, this had turned out to be a busy social season. I could sit home and feel sorry for myself and nurse my neck in private, missing what promised to be a wonderful weekend. Or I could suck it up. Jennifer was right, I decided. So what if I didn't look picture perfect? It was more important to be present for friends and to make memories while I could.

For Jeff and Stephanie's rehearsal dinner, I came up with what I thought was a smart idea. I wrapped a chiffon scarf loosely around my raw throat. It wasn't much of a fashion statement, but it would spare me from grossing anyone out. I popped on Frenchie and held my head as high as a sore neck would permit. The party took place at another estate I was thrilled to visit, a place I had driven by and—house freak that I am—ogled in the past. Mar-A-Lago in Palm Beach was now owned by Donald Trump. In the 1920s, the mansion had been the private residence of cereal heiress Marjorie Merriweather Post. It was built of aged Italian stone with a tall tower overlooking both the ocean and Lake Worth. Walking through the main house on that chilly night, I was dazzled by the high, gilded coffered ceiling of the living room.

Due to the weather, dinner, planned to be served outdoors, was moved into the large new Grand Ballroom behind the mansion. The space was decorated with typical Trump bravado, including Louis XIV-style gold trim and crystal chandeliers.

Any trace of self-consciousness I felt vanished the instant I saw Norm. Jennifer had talked him into coming as well. A mutual friend who suffered from ALS, Norm could no longer move his arms or legs, nor speak. I'd guess most of us in that condition would have stayed home and ducked public scrutiny.

Not Norm. I was awed by the love and effort and will it must have taken him just to show up that night. Looking back, I believe some indomitable spirit inside him wanted to reconnect with old friends one last time.

With his aide standing next to him, Norm slumped, pale and hunched over, in his wheelchair. A navy blue blazer hung on his shrunken limbs. As other guests came up to him, I stood aside, thinking how merciful it is that we don't know what fate awaits us. I flashed back to a dinner party at Norm's lovely farm-colonial home in Bloomfield Hills, Michigan, a few years before. He guided us around the house, standing tall, pointing out his daughter's ribbons in horsemanship, praising his wife's decorating. He beamed over a rosy wall paint in one room, wood paneling in another. At dinner he sat up straight at one end of the mahogany dining table, describing each wine as it was poured, proud to have picked and to share the perfect accompaniment for every course.

Now, when others moved on, I approached him. I leaned down and laid my hand on his bony arm. I kissed his cool forehead and looked into his expressionless eyes.

"Norm," I said, "it took you even more courage than it took me to be here tonight."

From the way he gurgled, I knew he understood.

Days later, our brave friend died.

Back in our hotel room after the party, I removed the scarf from my neck. No matter how gently I pulled, the fabric tore shreds of skin and left rivulets of blood among the scabbed and oozing patches. As gruesome as my neck looked before, it looked worse now. But I thought about Norm's determination and about what Rick had said. The next night I pulled on Gertrude, shiny and full and fresh from the wig store salon. I wore a pink-and-white cardigan sweater that left my throat exposed. No one mentioned that part of me looked as though I had stumbled into a landmine. At one point, I apologized for my neck to a guest who had once been a fashion designer. She said,

"I thought you tie-dyed it to match your sweater." It was a great line. I still don't know if she was kidding.

I love weddings; they reaffirm the possibility of romance. I like to hold Burton's hand and remember our ceremony, though actually it was more comical than romantic as my young cousin, the flower girl, had a tendency toward flatulence. In recent years, couples often ask Burton to photograph their wedding. He spends those evenings making sure he shoots all the guests and often fills albums with his pictures and gives them to the newlyweds as a wedding gift. I miss holding his hand during those ceremonies but figure his snapshots will be appreciated enough to warrant my sacrifice.

This wedding took place at the posh Everglades Club. White chairs were set up on the lawn of an interior courtyard ringed by columns of white marble. I always arrive early enough to secure an aisle seat with a clear view of the bride as she enters. Stephanie was a vision in an ecru gown with a café-au-lait sash. She wore a long veil of aged lace which Jennifer, in convincing me to come, had told me was first worn by Jeff's great-grandmother and later by his mother. The bride's father, Steve, an outgoing man we'd met the night before, also suffered from a form of ALS, although his case was less severe than Norm's. To escort his daughter down the aisle, Steve propelled himself in his motorized wheelchair, looking happy and not at all self-conscious.

After dinner, I witnessed another moment so filled with grace that I temporarily forgot all about my raw neck and my uncertain future. The band leader announced the bride's dance with her father. Stephanie glided onto the empty parquet floor and waited as her father zigged and zagged his wheelchair in time to the music. The grin on his face was almost as wide as the drum on the stage. When Steve stopped, his daughter bent down, flipped back the pedals of his chair, and gently helped him to a standing position. The bride's mother and the groom's mother and stepfather stood poised at the edge of the dance floor, ready to rush in if rescue were needed. I could feel everyone in the room holding their breath.

Stephanie placed her father's arms around her waist and wrapped her arms around him. Together, they swayed to the music for several seconds before Stephanie eased her father, still beaming, back into his chair. The band played "Unforgettable."

Back in Detroit, purple crocuses began poking their heads through stubborn, hard dirt. This joyful whisper of spring inspires any Midwesterner. But this year, Burton didn't seem as buoyant as usual. Over the past late summer, fall and winter, he had been strong when he needed to be strong. During my diagnosis, surgeries, chemo and radiation, he did the research, made the decisions and remained upbeat. Lately, I began to see deeper furrows in his forehead, to hear a flat tone in his voice. He walked with a tired step. He seemed to have given in to a depression he'd held off for months, months when he needed to stay positive for me. When you've known someone for almost forty years, you learn how to cope with their slumps. I had found I couldn't talk him out of those spells. When a bad mood overtook my husband, I had learned to give him time and space to work through it.

Occasional small pains still darted through my pelvis. Not enough to stop what I was doing, but enough to notice. The left side of my pubic bone throbbed. This had happened before, and Dr. Malone had told me not to worry. "After what you've been through, I'm not surprised," he said. This time the twinges seemed stronger, harder to put out of my mind, though they ceased after several seconds.

I didn't want to tell Burton about my symptoms. While the last nine months had been hard on both of us, I felt as though I was getting my life back. My treatment was finished, God willing, for good. My throat looked badly sunburned but I could hide most of the redness with concealer. My hair was developing a spiky attitude. I was organizing a birthday luncheon for my sister.

Burton had planned a hunting trip with some buddies. I hoped the getaway would cheer him up. He needed the time off. He had left me for exactly one night since my diagnosis, the night of Brenda's angel cards, and only because Brenda agreed to stay. I wanted him to go. I knew he wouldn't leave if he thought anything were wrong with me.

He asked how I was feeling. I'm a lousy liar.

"Call the doctor."

Dr. Malone said my twinges probably came from post-surgical scarring. He told me to come back and see him if the pain became recurring. Burton left town as planned, and I did my best to believe in the post-surgical scarring theory. When people asked how I felt, I smiled and said, "Great!" But in spite of a battery of Godsigns to reassure me, with each twinge, I wondered.

Time away improved Burton's spirits. He'd had a great time, he said. He'd enjoyed hanging out with the guys. They played Texas Hold 'Em, and he won.

"How do you feel?" he asked.

"Fine," I said. "Except for the weakness in my groin."

"Is it better or worse?"

"Hard to say."

If I elaborated on the soreness in my pubic bone, Burton would urge me to call the doctor again and to take another test, and it felt like I had already been subjected to enough radiation to destroy Hiroshima. A full set of CT scans had shown clear a month ago, and I had called Dr. Malone only days before. Instead of voicing my worries, I wrote about them. I decided to chart the throbbing for a few days, to see if there was a pattern.

The next day I sat at my desk. The pain in my pubic bone had not returned. Still, an uneasiness lay just below the cheerful surface of my morning. I opened my *Back from Betrayal* email account. I continued to receive and answer readers' messages. Two days before, Joann had sent me a forward. The subject line read "St. Therese's Prayer." Depending on how many emails I receive in a day, I often delete forwards without looking at them.

In this case, I tried to open the attachment but was unable to. I wrote back telling her so and thanked her for trying.

Psychologist and author Jeff Vezina analyzes synchronicity in his book *Necessary Chances*. He writes, "To approach synchronicity, we must learn to tolerate uncertainty and let ourselves be moved by the mysteries of the unlikely."

The next morning, shadowed by uncertainty and still worried about my pubic bone, I noticed another email from Joann. I had received Godsigns while in a labyrinth, a car, a theater, a pub. I had received them walking a beach and lying in bed. This was the first one I received through email.

Joann wrote, "You were so kind to me when I really needed understanding and words of wisdom. I thought it was worth typing this prayer to you." I have since learned there is uncertainty over the author of the prayer. It is attributed to St. Teresa of Ávila, to St. Thérèse of Lisieux, to Mother Teresa. I don't know which is correct. I had never heard the prayer before, but I was so grateful, at that moment, to read it.

Joann had gone out of her way to type the message I read below. When I reached the last lines, I drew in my breath.

> ... May you be content knowing you are a child of God.
> Let this presence *settle into your bones*, and allow your soul the freedom to sing, dance, praise and love.

CHAPTER 15

Still at the Party

There are only two ways to live your life. One is as though nothing is a miracle. The other is as if everything is.

—**Albert Einstein**

MELISSA ETHERIDGE, ALSO diagnosed with cancer the year before, appeared at the Grammy awards ceremony in full make-up and bald head. She sang "Piece of my Heart," a tribute to Janis Joplin, also a nonconformist, and ahead of her time, fashionwise. Joplin was one of the first to wear tattoos and feathers in her hair. As for Etheridge's lack of hair, I admired her courage in showing up the way she did. Now I had to choose.

As the date of the annual Karmanos fundraising dinner drew near, the pain in my pubic bone thankfully seemed to subside. I had a welcome new challenge: what to wear. A year before I had purchased a pale-blue beaded sweater and matching silk skirt. I was pleased to debut them. Long ago I learned not to wait for a special occasion to buy special-occasion clothes or risk becoming desperate at the last minute and settling for something I didn't adore.

The question was my hair. I had tried to love the dark stubble that peeked from my skull. I told myself I looked edgy. I admired the curve of my occipital bone. But I was no Melissa

Etheridge. I felt better in my wig. On the other hand, showing up with my scalp "au naturel" might make others struggling with cancer treatment feel more comfortable.

Brenda had supervised the color and cut of my wig. She had held my hand and cried with me on the day my head was shaved. More than half a year later, my voice quavered on my girlfriend's answering machine. "This may be the hardest fashion question I've ever asked you."

Brenda called back. "You are not your hair. You are not your wig. Are you going to wear make-up? A pretty dress? Wear whatever makes you feel good."

Shortly before the Karmanos event, I glanced at a leaflet that accompanied the invitation. Several items had been donated, including one from Tiffany—a slender gold cuff of small rosettes. I enjoy meaningful souvenirs, lasting objects to celebrate special occasions. We have purchased paintings or a new car or built a deck to mark different anniversaries. The Karmanos annual dinner was a big-time special occasion. The bracelet would make a fine memento of the evening—my chance to officially thank the hospital that had done so much for me. It would be a present to myself, honoring all that I had been through. I decided to bid on it, hoping it would not go for too high a price.

I reread the information to learn details of the auction. To my dismay, I realized I had misunderstood. The bracelet was part of a raffle, not an auction. If I had read right in the first place, I wouldn't have dreamt of owning such a prize. I crumpled up the paperwork and threw it into a waste basket. It wouldn't do me any good. I never won raffles.

The annual dinner took place downtown at Ford Field, the indoor arena where the Detroit Lions played. Hundreds of guests milled around the terrazzo-floored lobby, chatting and sipping drinks. The noise level soared. Most guests wore big turquoise feathers pinned to gowns or sprouting from tuxedo-jacket pockets. The feathers showed they had bought $50 raffle tickets.

Burton asked if I wanted to participate.

"You bet," I said. The donation was for a good cause, and I'd be embarrassed to be seen without a turquoise feather. I had no hope that my luck might change.

I checked my evening bag. Lipstick, lip liner, reading glasses, index cards, a pen. I had been so busy thinking about my remarks that I had forgotten to bring money or to remind my husband to do so.

Luckily, Burton is conscientious about always having cash on him. He reached into his pocket and pulled out a $100 bill. "This is all I have."

"It'll do," I said. "You sign the tickets. You're luckier than I am."

We received two turquoise plumes. I pinned mine to my sweater.

During cocktails, I sipped from a glass of cabernet sauvignon, glad for the nerve-calming benefits. Someone came up to say hello and bumped my arm. I watched a red tidal wave surge over the rim of my glass and slosh a softball-sized stain across the front of my light-blue silk skirt. The woman who jostled me seemed horrified. "I'm so sorry," she said over and over. "This is your big night and look what I've done."

"After what I've been through, this is nothing," I said. And I meant it.

Most of the time I was in treatment, I shunned alcohol, except for a rare glass of red wine which I justified for its anti-oxidant benefits. Once I was declared "cured ... until proven otherwise," I allowed myself the luxury of drinking again. On this particular occasion, white wine or vodka or champagne would clearly have been the more sensible choice. If I had to have a drink, that is. Which, under the circumstances, I did.

At dinner, more than 700 guests sat in a huge seven-story atrium. On the main floor, rows of round tables for twelve extended back from the stage. Still more tables were set up overhead on the mezzanine. We were seated in front, near the stage, along with Andy and Amy and David and his then-girl-friend, Nadine.

Dick Purtan, a popular Detroit radio personality, married to an ovarian-cancer survivor, emceed. On stage during dinner, he drew names from a glass bowl filled with raffle tickets. The first item went to someone else. The second was the bracelet. I felt my heart quicken but reminded myself not to get my hopes up. Dick reached into a bowl, peered at the ticket, and announced, "Burton Farbman."

"Oh, my God!" I shrieked. I jumped from my seat, bouncing up and down.

"Nothing to it," Burton said, beaming as though we had just won the lottery.

A volunteer brought over a small, shiny turquoise box. I cradled it in my hand, then slid the bracelet over my wrist. It fit like Cinderella's slipper. I felt my heart float up, up past the crowd on the mezzanine, up to merge with the stadium lights overhead. A burst of insight popped in my head like the flash of a camera. A connection that had nothing to do with logic but everything to do with trust and hope. The bracelet was a symbol, a symbol of my uphill fight against cancer and the chance of victory. I thought to myself: If, against all odds, I can win the very piece I wanted tonight, maybe, somehow, just possibly I can also win my bigger battle.

Large screens flanking the stage featured blow-ups of people at the podium. Jinny and Don, and the other event chairs and Dr. Ruckdeschel all spoke. Dr. V., a beloved Karmanos doctor, was honored. Noise from the crowd in back and overhead drowned out most of what was said. As hard as I had worked on my remarks, I feared the acoustical system was defective and that I wouldn't be heard either.

Dick Purtan announced us. Burton escorted me to the stage and returned to his seat. Standing at the microphone, I was relieved to hear the room fall silent. I raised my arm to show off my new bracelet and gave a royal wave. The audience cheered.

"I'm honored to be here tonight," I said. "I'm honored to be *anywhere* tonight."

Laughter rumbled through the audience. My heart fluttered. I had been heard.

"Will whoever was involved in my case please stand up? Doctors, nurses, technicians, family, friends? Whoever brought us chicken casseroles or made cabbage soup or left eyebrow pencil at my door?"

I had practiced my remarks and brought an outline. I didn't need it. I had lived what I wanted to say. Several years before, at a class I attended in public speaking, an instructor revealed that most peoples' biggest fear, even greater than dying, is public speaking. She told us to take advantage of every chance we got to speak publicly. "You never know what it will bring," she said. She also counseled, "Be yourself." I had taken her advice. I learned not to be self-conscious but rather to focus on reaching others. I taught the lessons to our sons, both of whom turned into fine public speakers. Sometimes our audiences are just family. When one of us has a birthday, we go around the table toasting the celebrant. Even our sons' old girlfriends got drafted to give toasts. The only time I was ever terrified to speak publicly was our *Oprah* appearance. I suffered my first-ever panic attack a few days before. But the speaking experience I'd had must have helped. On the set, I thought I sounded moronic. When the show ran, I was relieved to see I actually seemed rational.

When I asked people to stand that night, the lights shining on the podium were too bright for me to see into the audience, but I heard many chairs scrape the floor. I knew that dozens of people stood. They included Dr. Malone and Tina, his assistant; Dr. Forman and Denise and other radiation technicians; Dr. Ruckdeschel, the head of Karmanos; and Lynn Sinclair, who shepherded us through. I knew they included Dr. Jacobs, my throat surgeon; and nurses from the blood labs and chemo department. And Sara and Jenny, who took turns helping me at home. And Burton's executive assistant, Denise, who arranged appointments and wrote thank you notes. I knew they included Neal, who helped us figure out a diagnosis. And Brenda, who pulled me through so many meltdowns. And my sons, whose presence brought me such hope. And many other friends.

"You are all my angels," I said. "You in the medical field are also the angels of countless Karmanos patients. Past, present and future. All of you who are guests tonight are our angels as well because in being here you help fund the work of this fine medical center.

"Karmanos works miracles. I am one of those miracles. Last July, I was diagnosed with metastasized uterine cancer. Stage four. I thought my life was over. I would never have another chance to walk the woods up north with my husband. I wouldn't get to hear my new granddaughter's voice. Or go to lunch with my girlfriends again.

"But my family wouldn't let me give up. My friends wouldn't let me give up. God wouldn't let me give up. And Dr. Malone and Dr. Forman and Dr. Ruckdeschel said they hoped to cure me. So I had to fight. And over the past ten months, I kept fighting. I slogged through three surgeries. Six courses of chemo. Fifty-six rounds of radiation. And yes, it was rough. But I put on my wig and kept going. And here I am tonight. Still in my wig. And still at the party.

"Lance Armstrong disputes those who say he beat cancer. He writes, 'I didn't beat cancer. The doctors beat cancer. The medicine beat cancer. I survived cancer.'

"I hope to say the same thing. So far, thank God, I can.

"In the meantime, last weekend in the woods up north, I hunted for morels with Burton. Several weeks ago, I heard my granddaughter call my son 'Dada.' And three days ago, I shared hummus and tabouleh with some of my girlfriends to celebrate my birthday. A birthday I feared would never happen."

Ending my remarks, I thanked the audience for helping Karmanos continue to save the lives of countless patients, including mine.

You can tell when an audience supports you. You can feel it in the stillness, in the laughter, in the energy of the crowd. I felt grateful to have reached them. I left the stage to such an enthusiastic applause that, for an instant, I felt like Sally Field accepting the Oscar. They really liked me.

Later in the evening, a woman introduced herself and told me how she, too, had been treated at Karmanos and how grateful she was to still be alive. She wore a strapless green gown and pointed to the half-inch, white, raised chemo-port scar in her upper left chest. I drew the neck of my sweater aside and showed her mine. Part looked like hers, where the port had entered. The lower part, where the port came out, was arrow-shaped and pinker. We were like Girl Scouts admiring each other's merit badges.

When a horse is bitten or cut, its flesh grows back darker and raised. The term for such scars is "proud flesh." The poem, "For What Binds Us," captures the way I imagine most survivors feel about their scars. Poet Jane Hirshfeld writes, "All flesh is proud of its wounds, wears them as honors given out after battle ... "

At one point in the story of Peter Pan, Tinker Bell loses confidence. Her light starts to flicker out. To save her, Wendy and Peter Pan and the Lost Boys clap their hands and repeat, "I believe in fairies." When I was diagnosed, my light flickered, too. But there were people who believed in medicine. And believed in miracles. And believed in me even when my faith faltered. Doctors. Nurses. Radiation techs. Family. Friends. And most of all—my husband, my champion. Some of those people were our guests that night. Others had paid $350 a ticket to be there. Their belief made all the difference.

The next morning I lay in bed recalling the night before. I thought about the friends who had shown up or taken ads in the program. About the generous full-page ad my sister and mother had contributed. About the fun we'd had dancing, the survivors who had come up to share their stories and hugs.

With Mishe Bear tucked under my right arm and several more stuffed teddy bears, recent gifts, watching from a shelf across the room, I lifted my left hand off the ivory wool blanket. I pivoted my wrist back and forth. Tiny shards of golden light shone from delicate spirals. I had slipped the bracelet on the night before and hadn't taken it off. I hadn't told anyone that I wanted it. I didn't dare let myself dream it might be mine.

More than 700 people had attended the gala. We could purchase only two raffle tickets. I seldom cared about winning raffles. Generally the prize was a purse that a store had donated because it hadn't sold or an outfit that wouldn't fit. Or a china figurine or a vase I didn't want—something that would take up space, and as you've gathered, I was particular about what took up space in my home. If the prize had been cash, I'd have just donated it back to the charity anyway. But the night before was different. The night before I had longed for a simple, little, gold cuff bracelet. The night before, I, (or technically Burton, who did have a history of winning, and once, early in our marriage when we seriously needed the money, won $1,000 in a Mobil Oil instant-winner contest), had scored the very prize for which I yearned. I didn't own a lot of jewelry. I still wore the diamond Burton gave me thirty-nine years before. The oval center and side stones were originally set in platinum. To present it to me, Burton hid it in a Cracker Jack box. I had since had the stones inserted into a more contemporary, domed gold setting. I wore it every day. Except for that one ring, if I'd had a vault full of gems, I'd have traded them all for the simple gold cuff I'd won the night before. For what it signified to me.

I recalled the name Tiffany's had given my newest Godsign, and I shivered. The Rosebud Bracelet. God sent me roses.

Linda, a nurse with Dr. Brownstein, my holistic doctor, was a devout Christian. She spent her spare time reading the Jewish Torah and *Kabbalah*. She believed that deepening her knowledge of the Old Testament would enhance her understanding of the New.

Every few weeks, I visited Dr. B. for what he called an auto-vaccine treatment. My blood was drawn and spun on a machine which separated lighter-weight cells into a serum. The serum was then spun on another machine along with some of the cancer slides I brought with me each time. The process aimed to imprint cellular information, to create a new and informed serum. The informed serum was injected into three or four points in the lymph glands on the inside of my forearm to alert my immune system to guard against the troublemaking cells. "It's an approach used long before antibiotics were developed," Dr. B. said. "I don't know if it will help. In any case, it won't hurt to stimulate your immune system."

Waiting in one of Dr. B's small rooms, I sat on a paper-covered examining table chatting with Linda. Normally, she shared her newest bible studies with me. Now I told her about my latest Godsign. I held out my arm.

"They're rosebuds," I said. "God sent me roses."

She took my hand and turned it back and forth. "Have you counted them?"

"No," I said, and I did. "Twenty-six."

"I wonder what that means."

"Two plus six makes eight," I chirped. "Eight is my lucky number."

"But I wonder what it means in religious terms. You know numbers are important in the Old Testament."

"I know that. Funny it took a Christian to remind me."

That night, game six of the 2005 NBA Finals took place. The Detroit Pistons were playing the San Antonio Spurs. Our team hadn't won a game in Texas in eight years. Burton was away for the evening. I wouldn't normally watch a sports event by myself, but I was the mother of athletes, and this was an occasion. Sitting in bed, I picked up the remote control and turned on the TV. The game appeared on my first try. Technology was not my strength. Usually I'd rather read than watch television anyway. Our TV was complicated and often required two gadgets to operate. Sometimes Burton left a DVD movie in, and I couldn't figure out how to get the screen back to television mode though my husband had shown me several times. Sometimes I couldn't find one of the gadgets and would give up and wait for Burton to return. But this night I prevailed.

The previous game was played at The Palace, our home court. 22,000 fans in red, white and blue screamed and waved and carried on as if nothing—not the recent tsunami in Indonesia nor the reelection of George W. nor even the cancellation of the entire NHL hockey season—not a single thing mattered more than getting that ball through the hoop. Sports have a way of returning pride to a city that has lost so much. Detroiters love their teams and let them know it. Still, we lost.

I turned on the game just as the Pistons ran onto the SBC Center court. Despite the death march played on the loudspeaker, our team appeared determined. Some 19,000 spectators wearing black, white and silver roared and stomped against us, encouraged by a bevy of busty cheerleaders flinging their hair about. Despite the hostile atmosphere, the Pistons played with focus and resolve. They darted and dodged and flew and threw as if their lives depended on it and won the game by a miraculous nine points. Final score: 95-86. For more than two breath-suspending hours, I was too busy cheering and pumping my arms and phoning my sons to notice a single pelvic twinge.

After the game, a reporter asked guard Chauncey Billups how the Pistons had prevailed under such challenging conditions. "If it ain't rough, it ain't right," he said. I didn't cry when David sprained his ankle in tennis or Andy got knocked down in a football game. But cancer increases your sensitivity, and you don't know what will affect you. Chauncey's words about the Pistons' fight reminded me of my own. My eyes filled with tears.

Before turning off the light, I looked through the shelves in our library. I pulled out a book I had acquired during our marriage crisis, a period when I also sought help wherever I could find it.

Kabbalah, or Jewish mysticism, seeks to explain the relationship between an infinite, eternal creator and His mortal, finite universe. It proposes secrets God supposedly revealed to Adam. Early Kabbalistic documents date back to the first century A.D.

In *The 72 Names of God*, scholar Yehuda Berg writes about the significance of numbers in the Old Testament. A system called *Gematria*, from the ancient Greek word for geometry, interprets Hebrew words based on the numerical values of letters. The Torah mentions God's name 72 different ways. Each name has a numerical equivalent. Each number has a meaning. Rabbi Berg says if we are guided to a certain number, we should pay special attention to its meaning.

Back in bed, I turned to the page describing Name 26. It consists of three Hebrew letters: *Hei, Alef, Alef*. The letters read from right to left. *Hei* looks like a tiny two-legged table with the left leg not quite tall enough. *Alef* resembles a capital N with a gap below the right serif. *Hei* is the fifth letter of the alphabet; *Alef* is the first. Five, plus one, plus one equals seven. The translation of Name 26: Order from Chaos.

Reading on, I felt synapses spark in my brain. Name 26 carries special significance, Rabbi Berg writes. Of the ten dimensions (*Sefirot*) that form reality, the highest are called the Upper Three. God (*Ein Sof*) dwells at the top. The Upper Three exist outside our physical reality. The Lower Seven interact with our physical world. This is why the number seven turns up so often. Seven colors of the spectrum. Seven notes of the musical scale. Seven seas. Seven major continents. Seven days in a week. Seventh day of rest.

The 72 names of God are used as tools for meditation. Rabbi Berg concludes his discussion of each name with a suggestion for how to meditate upon it. When I read his meditation for Name 26, a charge buzzed around my rib cage. "Harmony always underlies chaos. With this Name, balance and serenity are restored among the seven days of the week. Order emerges from chaos."

The meditation seemed to be created just for me. Gazing at the Hebrew letters, I traced my fingers over them. Electricity tickled my fingertips. Chaos was a word I had used to describe my cancer experience. The chaos of working through confusing symptoms and reaching a diagnosis. The chaos that treatment imposed on my schedule and my spirits. The chaos of machines and chemicals that destroyed healthy cells along with malevolent ones. Contemplating Rabbi Berg's meditation, I took a few centering breaths and felt my shoulders lower. I prayed that balance, serenity and good health would return to my life. That order would indeed emerge from chaos.

Thinking about this extraordinary new Godsign, my mind skipped back to the one other time I received a hopeful message in numbers. It was several weeks before, on a day I felt especially low. I had undergone thyroid surgery. Soon after, I returned to gloomy Detroit from sunny Sarasota for five more weeks of radiation. I had stopped my car behind a rusty old Ameritech truck when I noticed the license plate: 8585MD. My lucky number and Burton's, combined with the medical abbreviation. Einstein said, "I am convinced that God does not play dice." To me, that license plate meant more than a roll of dice. It meant we were on the right road.

I don't understand how Godsigns happen—whether by design or by chance. I only know that when they occur, they can bring us hope. If we overlook or ignore the message, we are poorer for it. Godsigns are mysteries beyond human understanding. A force clever and powerful enough to create gravity or grandchildren or to part the Red Sea was surely capable of planting a message on a license plate and putting it in front of the one person in the universe who needed to see it at that moment.

Trying to grasp the mathematical probability of my license plate discovery, I turned to Wikipedia, my online bible. "A mathematical coincidence can be said to occur when two expressions show a near-equality that lacks direct theoretical explanation." The probability was no clearer. I just shook my head.

Although I can add and subtract, I have never been adept with numbers. Give me a story problem about Jenny who has $50 to spend, and shoes cost $20 and blouses, $25, and how many items can she afford, I find myself thinking about the heel of the shoe or the ruffle on the blouse instead of the computation. I am even more baffled by complicated equations with ratios and tangents and cosines. But those who excel at numbers claim that there is a purity, a perfection to mathematics.

Now, sitting in bed, marveling at the wisdom of Name 26, I realized something humbling. In spotting that license plate, I had not looked deep enough. There was a meaning more profound than the presence of our lucky numbers, which caught my attention in the first place. The universe had tried to give me a message with even greater significance. How many others might I have missed?

Contemplating Name 26, I happened to add up the numbers on the license plate I had seen a few weeks before. My arms broke out in goose bumps.

On a hot July afternoon up north, I made cups of green tea, poured the amber liquid over ice and added a squeeze of lemon and a squirt of agave nectar. It had taken me several weeks to stop craving sugar. I rarely ate desserts any longer, although four days earlier I had savored a bite of my granddaughter's first birthday cake.

That morning I shot 56 for nine holes. Until the past year, such a score might have drawn some less than lady-like assessment from my lips. Now the sheer ability to walk nine holes, regardless of my score, pleased me. I was overjoyed to have my energy, and my life, back. My pelvic twinges were less frequent. When they occurred, I described them in my journal and tried to forget about them.

A few weeks had passed since I discovered the significance of Name 26, Order from Chaos. Burton and I sat on the porch of our farmhouse sipping iced tea. We talked about how almost a year had passed since my diagnosis.

"I gave you quite a challenge," I said.

"There were some pretty tense times," Burton said. "But it looks like we've dodged a bullet."

I knocked my knuckles on both temples then folded my hands at my chest and bowed my head in gratitude for all the forces that helped me to survive.

"I would never, ever call cancer a gift. But real gifts came with it," I said. "The ability to better appreciate the moment. More compassion. Less negative thinking. A closer relationship with you and the kids."

"And God."

I nodded. "And Godsigns."

"What was the date of your diagnosis?"

"I don't know," I said. "It was right after Shelley and Richard's party."

Shelley, my friend with the sexy, black leather jacket and the vein-stripping doctor, spent summers in a pretty white house surrounded by gardens bursting with pink roses. In another life, I had featured the residence in *Better Homes and Gardens*. The house overlooked Round Lake in downtown Charlevoix. The previous summer, Shelley and Richard had hosted a big party in their terraced backyard during Venetian Weekend. Venetian Weekend was an annual festival in Charlevoix that took place the last weekend in July. It included a carnival where, as youngsters, our boys enjoyed riding the loop-de-loop and tossing bean-bags at bottles to win chartreuse-green stuffed snakes and feasting on cotton candy. It included a boat parade and a loud and dramatic fireworks display. I remembered boats circling the harbor below, festooned with colorful lights. I remembered a warm night, cherry pies, a cake decorated with red, white and blue sprinkles, curlicues of light exploding in the dark sky and whistling down to the lake. I remembered returning to Detroit the next day, driving to a clinic the morning after, praying my way through a pelvic MRI. I remembered how, an hour later, I sat in my internist's office and heard the word everyone fears. I didn't remember the date.

"I'll check," I said. I got up from the porch swing and padded, barefoot, into our bedroom. My 2004 date book sat in a drawer of the desk on my side of the bed. Unlike many of my friends, I hadn't graduated to the trendier Filofax in a jazzy-colored leather binder or, more recently, to some high-tech electronic device. As averse to change as I am, I had used the same old-fashioned appointments book for over three decades, procuring a new one each fall for the following year. It was a decidedly-un-chic DayMinder, covered in black plastic, with a metal spiral binding and the year engraved in silver on the front. I needed one page a day to pen in social dates, tee times, my grocery list, errands, phone calls, birthdays—the major and minor stuff that makes up a life. The stuff I could now, joyfully, record again. I pulled my old date book out of the drawer and flipped to the page for the last Monday in July. I put my index finger on the date and blinked several times to be sure I was seeing right.

There's a Yiddish expression that sums up the sense that anything is possible, no matter how unlikely, whether we understand it or not. *Klyne velt, groyser Gott.* The world may be small, but God is big.

Most of us learn the hard way. Illness is one of the hardest. It is a cruel teacher, but an effective one. Letting go of fear and staying in the moment are delicate sprouts. They take a lot of tending and are easily trampled by old attitudes and habits. I prayed I had learned the lessons I needed. I prayed I wouldn't have to spend any more anguish relearning them. Considering the challenges of aging, and the unpredictability of health, I imagined I would.

I still ponder what my disease meant and why I had to go through something so tough. Why Patsy and Jackie and too many other friends lost their battles. Why my mother took such punishment and my father suffered such pain. The best answer I have heard to such inexplicable questions came from an eight year old.

I was in my forties when Dad died. He and Mom had divorced a few years after he turned Catholic. He later married a Catholic woman with whom he spent many happy years. When I accompanied Margaret, Dad's widow, to the funeral home, I made a suggestion. I had once attended a wake for a Protestant who was an avid tennis player and had run a large ad agency in Detroit. He lay in state holding his favorite tennis racquet in his hands. As we waited to see the funeral home director, I suggested to Margaret that Dad, a devoted golfer, might be buried holding his putter. Margaret's emphatic "*No!*" was underscored by widened, greenish-brown eyes and contracted brow. When I arrived at the visitation, I understood. As Dad lay in a coffin, his hands clasped a rosary. A cross adorned the white satin lining inside the lid of the open casket. Horrified would be too strong a word for my reaction; uncomfortable wouldn't be strong enough. Instead of guiding visitors to view the body, I hovered in the anteroom. A priest conducted the service at a Catholic church. Dad was buried in a Catholic cemetery.

At the reception at Dad and Margaret's home, a member of their prayer group came up to me. Thelma was someone I knew and liked. She asked how I was.

I said, "I'm having a hard time with the Catholic thing."

"Let me tell you a story," Thelma said. Recently she was babysitting for her grandsons. She took them to the swimming pool at her condo in Florida. Five-year-old Peter looked into the water and asked why he could see himself. His eight-year-old brother, Stephen, compared the water to a mirror. Peter frowned and shook his head. A nearby adult made an attempt. He explained the principle of specular reflection, how an incoming and outgoing ray make the same angles in respect to a surface.

Peter's forehead remained wrinkled. He pointed at the water. "But why am I there?"

Stephen tried again. He said, "Don't you see, Peter? It's a mystery."

"Peter's face broke into a smile," Thelma said. "He nodded his head and said, 'Ah, a mystahwee!'"

She took my hands and gazed at me. Creases winged from her compassionate blue eyes. "There are things we will never understand," she said. "It's okay to let them remain a mystery."

The date I first learned I had cancer: July 26th. 7/26.

On August 8th, I wondered if I'd receive a Godsign. The date was my lucky number, doubled. It was a day in which the temperature also reached double eights and I slathered on SPF 30 suntan lotion. In shorts and t-shirts, Burton and I strapped our bikes with bungee cords to the Four Winns Funship we shared with our sons. The bow had just enough room for two bikes. We headed north on Lake Charlevoix and west on adjoining Round Lake through the harbor. We glanced up at our old home, grey vinyl-sided with white trim and a wraparound porch. It now belonged to Andy and Amy. I loved that house and was glad it was still in the family. We passed the Sitners' house next door, the one that earned me the cover of *Better Homes and Gardens*. And the Ramseys' old house, and Shelley and Richard's as well.

Burton steered through the channel to Lake Michigan and then revved the engine. We sped across Traverse Bay to Harbor Springs. Tying down the boat at a marina, we raced away on our bikes before anyone discovered we lacked permission to dock there. We rode to L'Esprit, one of my favorite antique shops, then to Turkey's Café for lunch. After, we biked along the edge of Lake Michigan, admiring stately homes that rose on money-green lawns, accented with wide front porches, columns and window boxes blooming with red and coral geraniums. It was a lovely day, a day I appreciated all the more for the pure joy of being on a bike instead of an examining table. But no Godsign.

When the wind picked up, we returned to our boat. It bobbed, unnoticed, where we'd left it. We strapped the bikes back down and made a clean getaway. Burton switched the radio to a fifties station and I belted out lyrics to "Running Bear" and "Rock Around the Clock". As the boat bounced through sparkling blue water, "Let's Twist Again" began to play. Burton idled the engine in the middle of the bay. We danced, laughing and gripping the captain's chair or the gunnels to steady ourselves as we swiveled our hips and tried to bend knees that did not flex as easily as they had almost fifty years before when we learned to twist. Our spirits hadn't rusted as badly as our joints.

Back at the dock in Charlevoix, Burton helped me off the boat. The low water level rendered stepping up to the dock a considerable stretch, but one I could again manage comfortably. I sat on the dock while Burton snapped on the canvas covers, a job I left to him to spare my fingernails. The old me would not have wasted time. I'd have skimmed a magazine or cleaned out my handbag or made a cell-phone call while I waited. The new me gazed at an American flag, rippling against the cloudless sky, and watched seagulls glide and listened to the water lapping.

And then I spotted them. Not one, but two Godsigns waiting to be noticed. The name of the boat docked directly across from ours: "In The Game." I said a prayer of thanks that I still was. Four slips away, I noticed a larger boat. Spelled out in capital letters, the name of that boat represented a lesson I'd learned over and over during the past year and would spend the rest of my hopefully long-and-healthy life continuing to learn: PATIENCE.

I spent many years trying to eradicate fear from my psyche. I've finally realized it can't be done. Fear has been hard-wired into our brains since cavemen dodged giant lizards. The best I can do is to go easy on myself. To feel the fear, accept it as normal and natural, and try to let it go. Some days I let go better than others. On those days I manage to replace fear with hope. Hope is hard-wired into us, too.

It took many friends, shrinks and self-help experts to help me understand the best antidote to fear. It is a lesson easily said and more easily forgotten. There is a secret to living peacefully, to settling my turbulent mind, to reeling it back in from my tendency to catastrophize. It is focusing on the moment, reveling in it. It is relaxing into, not railing against, what happens. Taoists call this *Wu-Wei*, the principle of nonresistance, of swimming with the current.

Cancer hones your appreciation of everyday marvels. You count them in small moments. The chance to have your granddaughter hold your finger and escort you to her playroom. The tart crunch of a honey crisp apple, the glory of a Mason jar spilling over with cosmos, the whisper of rain, the miracle of riding a bike. Each moment presents a chance for humble gratitude, for staying in the now.

I do a gratitude list at least once a day. At first, I wrote the list in my journal. Now, when I pray, I thank God for the many things that are right about my life, and I specify several of them. As busy as God is, I figure He appreciates knowing He has happy customers. To have healthy children and grandchildren, to live in America, to have a home and food on the table and a loving family and friends—these alone are off-the-charts blessings.

I am grateful for my husband's willingness to take over. My case was confusing and frightening. On top of the physical toll of cancer and its treatment, having to pursue the research and consider the possibilities and make the decisions would have been more than I could handle. I'd have spent all my energy second-guessing myself. Burton's taking on the medical role gave me the chance to focus on my spiritual side, a side I consider equally important in fighting any disease. It also helped to further heal our relationship.

I am grateful, too, for the Godsigns that helped lighten my fears. At a time when I struggled against the awfulness of what was happening to me, the universe sprinkled down a series of little miracles. Right or wrong, I saw them as God's way of cheering me on. Of letting me know something bigger was in charge. That things would be okay, no matter the outcome. Godsigns helped when I needed help. They nudged my attention back into a healthier mindset. That was good enough for me.

For more than a century, modern science has tried to prove or disprove or understand anecdotal phenomena. The problem with such testing is the mind that perceives Godsigns differs from our everyday mind, which is trained to be logical and linear. Modern science would no doubt pooh-pooh any notion of signs generated by some larger universal force. Yet most people, scientists included, have had powerful experiences they can't explain or categorize.

Contemplating Godsigns reminds me of the question about the tree falling in the forest. The question implies that noise requires a listener. Likewise, an object or event needs a perceiver, an interpreter, to represent a Godsign. Over the years, hundreds of thousands of drivers probably followed or stopped behind that beaten up Ameritech truck. Thousands of them may have noticed the license plate and never given it a thought.

Godsigns cannot be generated at will. They cannot be forced. Part of their joy is their unexpectedness, their element of surprise. If we remain alert and open and ready to receive the mystery, I believe we will find it. And when it appears, it can, in that moment, bring hope or a message or redemption to our lives.

I look forward to every full moon. Each one marks a personal triumph. I feel as though the heavens have floated a big, golden balloon in celebration of my recovery and that of everyone else on earth who has experienced a narrow escape. Each full moon pays homage to God's amazing gifts. When I gaze upward, my heart swells with joy until it feels as full as the moon itself. I have lived to see another one.

I've become a devotee of the lunar cycle, also called the synodic period, which actually takes 29.5 days. To thank God for my recovery, Rabbi Cohen, the Orthodox rabbi with whom Burton studied while I was in treatment, introduced me to a new habit. When I see a full moon, I fold my hands at my chest, bow my head and murmur "*Baruch HaShem.*" The phrase translates to "Thanks be The Name," because Orthodox Jews do not speak the name of God outside of formal prayer.

One benefit of God's being invisible is perceiving Him as we wish. Not being Orthodox, I want to believe in a God with whom I can have an intimate relationship. A God I can call on in any circumstance. On a plane, on the street, in a car or bed or temple. Even on a golf course (although He isn't as cooperative as He could be in that realm). Some religions ascribe to a more demanding and punitive God. I prefer to believe in a compassionate and encouraging divine force. For me, God is a best friend, a moral guide, a motivator and a listener. He brings out the best in us. He *is* the best in us. And He can be infinitely creative in getting our attention.

Burton and I sometimes disagree on exactly when the moon turns full, but I believe I have the definitive eye for lunar phases. I am so grateful for each full moon that I start looking skyward two or three days ahead of time. I launch early *Baruch HaShems* during the waxing gibbous period, before the left edge puffs out and the entire sunlit part of the moon faces the earth, and the earth, moon and sun are aligned.

More conservative Jews observe *Rosh Hodesh*, the first day of the lunar month, a time to celebrate the survival of the Jewish people. The moon marks my personal *Rosh Hodesh*. It is a string around my finger, reminding me of how lucky I am to still admire it from the earth's perspective.

Author Joan Anderson ran away from her secure, familiar life, despite the risk to her marriage and the disapproval of others. She wrote about the experience with a candor and power that inspired me when completing my first book. More than two years before my battle with cancer, I read Anderson's *A Year by the Sea*.

Several months after my cancer treatment was finished, I noticed an announcement in a local newspaper up north. Joan Anderson would conduct a seminar nearby. The morning of the seminar, I trotted up our farmhouse stairs, grateful to once again mount steps without pain. I pulled Joan's book from a shelf, slipped it into my tote bag, climbed into the truck and headed for the Petoskey Middle School.

The workshop, held in the auditorium, was sponsored by the Northern Michigan Hospital Foundation. The audience turned out to comprise mainly oncology nurses, a breed of compassionate heroes I had grown to trust and admire. They looked so human and life-sized sitting in padded chairs, wearing slacks and sweaters.

Joan spoke about the need to nurture ourselves and receive love—lessons I had learned over and over during the past months. She asked us to think of a relative we admired and to name a trait which described that person. People called out adjectives. "Fun-loving." "Considerate." "Independent."

I thought about my husband and how, despite his ADD-driven disorganization, he tracked down doctors and kept after them and sent and received reports in pursuing my diagnosis and treatment. I thought about how he escorted me to countless appointments at any hour, never complaining. How he drove me to pick up a yogurt smoothie after each radiation treatment. And how he continued to hunt for approaches to alternative care. I called out: "Tenacious."

Joan wrote our words on the pad of paper on her easel. She said, "You value in others the same traits you have in yourself. Take a minute to appreciate how fun-loving, considerate, independent and tenacious you are." Audience members continued to call out traits, and Joan continued scribbling them down with her blue marker. "I'm going to add wild and salty," she said.

I attend book readings and authors' talks whenever I can. I love to hear someone read or discuss his or her own work. When I read a book, the author becomes my friend. Occasionally I'm disappointed that the writer is not as authentic or likable as he or she seemed on paper. Joan was exactly what I expected—open, funny, caring. I liked her as much in person as I did on the page.

During the break, I approached Joan and asked her to sign my copy of her book. I thanked her for the courage her memoir had given me and showed her a postcard featuring the cover of mine.

"My book came out last year," I said. "Since then, I celebrated my sixtieth birthday. My family was on *Oprah* four times. My first grandchild was born. And I fought stage-four cancer."

Joan's blue eyes opened wide. It was the first time I had seen her speechless all morning. "I need to give you a hug," she said. And she did. A full-chest contact, arms tight around me, honeysuckle-scented, feel good, energy-filled hug.

Then she stepped back. Her gaze drilled into mine.

"I have a question for you." She paused for a second, as though not sure how to phrase it. "How did you overcome your fear of dying?"

It was a profound, courageous question from someone I felt as though I knew but who had just met me. Memories came rushing back. The soreness of my so-called groin pull. The dread that flooded my gut the first time I heard the term "lesions." The sting of needles and radiation burns. The exhaustion of chemo. I tasted the metallic flavor of contrast dyes, smelled the worry that accompanied every CT scan. I felt the ache of not living long enough for my granddaughter to know and love me the way I knew and loved my grandmother. Of wondering if Burton might find someone else with whom to spend his old age.

But I stood in that auditorium and looked at this wild and salty woman and my voice barely shook.

"I don't know if I did overcome my fear of dying," I said. "I just focused on living."

Epilogue

CANCER OPENS YOUR arms to life. It heightens your awareness of colors and smells and sounds. It deepens your appreciation for big events and small gestures. It changes your mind.

I never wanted a surprise party. Over the years, I'd told Burton how I felt. If I were going to have a party, I wanted to look forward to it, to have my hair and make-up done, to wear something fabulous but not so trendy that, in years to come, it would look silly in photos. Burton respected my wish. Although he liked surprises, he never threw a surprise party for me.

Once you're hit with cancer, something you've perceived only from an abstract, safe distance gallops toward you, rears up and kicks you in the gut. You don't know how much time you have left. However much it is, you want to make the most of it. As she was dying, Erma Bombeck wrote a column, "If I Had My Life to Live Over." It still sometimes circulates on email. I reread it every time. She regretted how her faded sofa prevented her from inviting more guests to dinner, how worrying about her hairdo kept her from enjoying car rides with the windows down.

About two years after my treatment, I realized that on my death bed, I didn't want to look back and know I'd let a few strands of thin hair get in my way. "I may have changed my mind about not wanting a surprise party," I said to Burton. And then I forgot about it.

We spent the next winter in Sarasota, a glorious season of freedom. Definition: lots of golf and dinner dates and no doctors. We returned to Michigan in early May, three days before my sixty-fourth birthday. I had booked dinner with our children and now two granddaughters and a grandson for the next night. That morning, for my birthday present, Brenda came over to reorganize my closet.

"At our age, it's easy to look frumpy," Brenda said. She pointed to the jeans I was wearing—a little old, a lot worn, but comfortable. "Case in point."

"Got it," I said, not the slightest bit insulted. Brenda's word was usually gospel with me, but I was not about to give up my favorite pair of jeans. Maybe I'd retire them up north to the farm. In any case, I'd remember not to wear them around my best girlfriend.

In my closet, Brenda eliminated some things, re-combined others. She told me to update my wardrobe by acquiring pants that flared at the bottom and a white wash-and-wear shirt from Brooks Brothers. "You'll live in it," she promised. When it comes to clothes, Brenda has very definite opinions. But she is also tactful. Her unsolicited observation about my jeans was a rarity. Normally, she waited for me to ask if she approved of my choices. As an ex-fashion editor, I knew how fast styles changed. Since I no longer devoured magazines to keep current, I relied on Brenda. Even though she gave up her fashion career, she continued to comb websites and publications and stores and remained a fashion expert. She pulled out a black, knee-length pleated skirt and suggested I shorten it and wear it with black tights. She combined a chiffony floral skirt with a lavender jewel-neck cashmere sweater, a pashmina shawl and a pair of grey leggings. I owned the leggings as a result of a previous fashion foray with Brenda.

"At our age, we need to make an effort to look cute all the time," Brenda said. "For instance, what are you doing tonight?"

"Dinner at the club with the family."

Brenda's expression remained unchanged. She surveyed the jacket section of my closet with professional detachment and pulled out a new matte-gold leather jacket. "For tonight I like the jacket and grey flannel pants you bought the last time we went shopping." She combined the jacket and pants with a sexy, white tank top and sling-back pumps and hung the outfit on a hook in my closet.

"I love it," I said.

After my fashion guru left, I reconsidered. The outfit she picked for that night was fabulous, perfect for a glamorous party. But not for dinner with grandchildren. Brenda didn't have grandchildren or belong to the same country club. She didn't consider 3½-year-old Alexis and her 1½-year-old sister, Camryn. They were likely to fingerprint macaroni and cheese on my new jacket on our way to the potty or dessert table. If I wore something more practical, Brenda would never know.

That afternoon, my sister, Anne, and her husband, Mike, arrived from California on their way to New York. Anne asked what I was wearing that night.

"Good black jeans," I said. In recent years, the club had succumbed to contemporary fashion and changed its old anti-denim policy.

"I brought a dress," Anne said. "Why don't you step it up a little? I'd feel more comfortable."

"Okay," I agreed, deciding to humor her. I'd wear the lavender floral print skirt combination. It was cute enough for dinner out. Not fabulous, but nice. The skirt was a couple of years old, but the leggings updated it. And small fingerprints wouldn't show.

We were due at the club at 6:30. At 6:00, Anne—curvy in a black sheath—and Mike joined us in our library for a glass of wine. At 6:25, the phone rang. Burton spoke briefly to David. "Got it," he said. Hanging up, he launched into a story about a recent golf game. I realized it could take a while.

"Hon," I said, "Alexis and Camryn only have a few minutes of good behavior in them." I pointed to my watch.

Burton hates it when I point to my watch. He rolled his eyes and enunciated each syllable. "When I finish the story."

Ten minutes later, Burton finally sunk the putt on the 18th hole.

"Can we leave now?" I asked.

"After I go to the bathroom."

Burton has an iron bladder. Still, I thought nothing of his need to pee. Nor did I notice that he carried his cell phone into the powder room.

As we pulled up the driveway to Franklin Hills Country Club, I noticed that the parking lot overflowed with cars.

"It's busy tonight," I said.

"Sunday night dinners must be popular," Burton said.

We had joined this club early in our marriage. My parents and grandparents also belonged, which—as long as we weren't convicted felons—basically rendered our acceptance a slam dunk. In recent years, our sons had joined, too. Sunday night cookouts with our family were my favorite activity at the club, though I also enjoyed being able to play golf close to home. A requirement for membership was giving generously to the community, which took away part of the guilt I might otherwise have felt about belonging to a private club that excluded some applicants. Instead, as usual, I was just glad to be included.

Anne, Mike, Burton and I pulled up to the front of the Cotswold-style brown brick-and-stone clubhouse, designed by my great-uncle Albert. We were fifteen minutes late. The parkers greeted us. Ours was the only car in the circular driveway.

David met us at the door. He wore a blue chambray shirt with paisley-lined cuffs turned back. He was tanned from a tanning machine—something I repeatedly warned him against and he repeatedly ignored. I had to admit, the glow made him look movie-star handsome.

"Are you excited, Mom?"

"I'm always excited to see my family."

We walked past the sitting room off the front lobby. Walls were lined with photos of past presidents. Burton had been president here twenty-five years ago. I glanced at his photo, remembering how when he was president, I served as food chairperson—a vital position in a Jewish club as we Jews love our food. After club events, we often sent notes to the staff commending them on the food and service. When Burton retired, the staff did something they had never done before. Every employee signed a letter telling Burton how much they had enjoyed the year under his watch. I framed the letter and hung it on a wall in his office, along with several business awards and articles and a plaque with the ball from his hole-in-one. Of all the tributes on the wall, he was proudest of that letter.

As we turned to walk down the hall, we passed a plaque inscribed with the names of each year's womens' tennis champion. Amy's name was etched on small, brass plates for the several years she had won, which was any year she wasn't pregnant. I was proud to have a family of athletes, especially since the allotment of jock genes did not extend to yours truly.

The lights were low in the ballroom at the end of the Pewabic-tiled corridor. Pewabic Pottery was founded in Detroit in the early twentieth century at the height of the Arts and Crafts movement. Many of the tiles created there had a unique, lustrous glaze and were still prized in numerous Detroit private and public buildings. I admired their worn brown patina whenever I walked the floors of this clubhouse.

As we entered the ballroom, the lights in the big wrought-iron chandeliers popped on. The room was jammed with people, all of whom yelled a thunderous, *Surprise!*

I gasped and fell back against my husband, as though jolted by a sonic boom. I said, "Brenda's going to kill me."

Guests began pushing toward me. Andy and Amy held our granddaughters in their arms. Alexis and Camryn, in pretty, ruffled dresses, gave me hugs and were whisked away. I was clutching a Kids"R"Us plastic bag with camouflage-printed bikinis I'd brought back from Florida for our granddaughters. My girlfriend Sandy grabbed the bag from me so it wouldn't show in the video of the party. "Don't lose it," I called.

Brenda came toward me, gestured to my outfit, and laughed.

I shrugged. "Right as usual."

"At least you wore something I approved."

A number of guests were casual friends I hadn't seen in a few years, since before my book was published, because we were often away from Detroit. Many hadn't known how to react to a memoir about Burton's and my marital problems, and so they hadn't reacted at all. At least to me. I'm sure they had plenty to say to each other. An old friend Bonnie, among the guests that night, was one of the few who openly let her disapproval be known. Shortly after *Back from Betrayal* came out, Bonnie had run into Burton at Steve's Deli, our local hangout. She'd asked Burton how he could have allowed me to publish such a revealing book. Burton said, "Suzy's a writer." Bonnie said, "You should have given her an eraser."

Dozens of people came up to greet me. Men in dark suits. Women in sophisticated cocktail clothes—gold sequins, red silk, black lace, fancy jewelry—the dressy-chic look Brenda had encouraged me to wear.

Despite feeling a little like the country mouse, I had a magical night. More than 200 friends and relatives greeted and hugged me. Betsy, my best friend from high school, had driven more than four hours from Traverse City in northern Michigan. Since we were teenagers, we called each other Zeke.

"Zekey," she huffed, wrinkling her nose and pointing to my legs as though something creepy were crawling there. "What are those?"

"Leggings," I said. "A new trend."

"One that will never make it to Traverse City."

Burton had invited my entire medical team. Most of them came. Dr. Moss, the internist who first discovered my problem. Lynn Sinclair, who smoothed our way through the hospital system. Dr. Ruckdeschel, who oversaw my case. Dr. Jacobs, my throat surgeon. Dr. Forman, my radiologist.

Seeing Dr. Forman, tears I had fought back, welled up in my eyes. "If it weren't for you, I might not be here tonight."

"What do you mean, *might*?"

After dinner, David emceed a program. David has been a natural with a microphone since childhood. For the traditional candle-lighting ceremony of his Bar Mitzvah, I offered to help him write poems or introductions for the people invited to light a candle on his thirteenth birthday cake. Just give him the names, he said. He'd handle it. He had guests laughing over his escapades with longtime babysitter Sari Beth and crying over the recent loss of his grandmother, Edith. At my surprise party, he was just as funny and eloquent about me. My girlfriends Brenda, Peggy, Sandy, Sally, Ginny and Florine sang an original song about me. My sister wrote and sang a solo. Andy took the mic and said, "Mom always writes birthday poems for my brother and me. Tonight I wrote one for her." He read a clever poem.

The lights dimmed and a video appeared on a large screen. It showed pictures of me as a baby, a Brownie, a ballerina. It showed the family at our sons' graduations. It showed me at Meredith headquarters in Des Moines, Iowa, giving a thumbs-up as I stood in front of a blow-up of my *Better Homes and Gardens* cover shot. Family and friends talked about me. David spoke with my adorable, new grandson, Hunter, squirming on his lap. Alexis sang "Happy Birthday," blissfully off key. Burton spoke about the fun we'd shared, the pride we took in our family.

Still on screen, Burton said, "Suzy, ever since I've known you, you've wanted to write a book. You wrote hundreds of columns and articles, and they were always great. But you wanted to create something with more lasting value. You tried fiction but weren't comfortable with it. You didn't think your life was interesting or controversial enough for non-fiction. So I racked my brain and finally came up with a subject for you." On screen, he paused. A devilish smile crossed his face. "I don't expect you to thank me, but I did it for you." As my husband's words registered, the entire audience howled with laughter. I laughed as hard as anyone, realizing how far we had come, and how, in just a few words, Burton had brought humor to a very sensitive subject and how grateful I was to laugh again.

At the end of the video, our friend Eric from northern Michigan played his guitar and sang "Suzy Lights up the Town." The lights came back on, and I realized Eric was not singing on screen. He was standing a few yards from our table.

I got up and walked over to Eric. "Not yet," he said into the mic. But I was beside him, and his voice broke, and he couldn't finish singing. He embraced me instead.

After, Burton took the microphone. I stood beside him.

"Suzy and I have gone to lots of weddings where the newlyweds call each other soul mates and best friends for life," Burton said. "I always think: *What do they know? They haven't been tested.* When you've lived through forty-plus years with someone, you have faced adversities together. If you're lucky, you come out stronger for them. Then … " his voice broke, "you know what it means to have a best friend."

Burton's words caused a tingling from my scalp to my toes. I scanned the audience—children, relatives, friends—absorbing the love. I took the microphone from my husband.

"I couldn't have put it better, and I'm the writer in the family." I kissed Burton's soft lips. "Eric wrote the song he sang tonight for my sixtieth birthday. The first time he sang it, Burton and I were at our farmhouse up north with one other couple. I had just been diagnosed with cancer. I cried through every note. I wondered if I'd ever light up any place again. I'm thrilled to hear the song tonight under much better circumstances, surrounded by people I love."

I looked at my husband, who had gone through so much with me. We had grown up together, lived through joy and pain.

His black hair had turned silver since we met forty-three years before, but he still had the rosy cheeks and bedroom eyes I'd fallen for on our first date.

"Thank you for your amazing support. Thank you for contacting doctors around the world, some of whom are here tonight. For dragging me to countless appointments. For refusing to give up on me.

"I'm glad I changed my mind about never having a surprise party. This has been the party of my life. We did it, didn't we? We lit up this town tonight."

Elisabeth Kubler-Ross analyzes the typical stages of dealing with a crisis: denial, rage, bargaining, depression, acceptance. In looking back at my cancer ordeal, I see that I excelled at the first and the fourth stages. I spent many days denying what was obvious to others. And many of the weeks that followed, depressed. If I were better at rage, I might have been less inclined to internalize stress and might not have gotten sick in the first place. Bargaining is another underdeveloped skill, like paddling a canoe. I prayed my heart out that God would make me well but didn't figure I had anything significant enough to offer in return. I did keep thinking: *Better me than one of my kids,* but I don't think that qualifies as bargaining. I only shine at bargaining at an antiques show when I'm willing to walk away. If the vendor has a cute dog or has mentioned her handicapped child, I'm likely to settle for a higher price because I think she needs the money. So much for bargaining. Acceptance? Gifts that come with cancer, yes. Disease itself? No way.

Cancer doesn't play fair. It sneaks up when you're not looking. By the time you discover it, its tentacles are imbedded. Once you've been diagnosed with cancer, you remain on guard. Every new scan stiffens you with worry. When you read an obituary about someone who dies in her thirties or forties, you wonder why, and check to see if donations are suggested to the American Cancer Society, and sigh when they are. You smile at obituaries of people in their nineties. You wonder why some survive and others don't. You try not to spend too much time thinking about it. Because you don't want to tempt fate with bad thoughts. Or overly confident ones. Because you'll never know the answer. As long as you're on this side of the fairway, it will remain a "mystahwee."

There is awe and gratitude at having faced down a cancer diagnosis. I am stronger for it. "Strong" is shorthand for being dragged under by fear and flailing my way back to the surface to gasp for air again and again. I know cancer could recur or some other grim disease present itself. Puh, puh, puh! Spitting three times on your first and middle fingertips is a Jewish superstition to avoid bringing on the evil eye.

I wake up at night and feel a sensation in my pelvis. My mind strains to remember: Have I felt this before? Is this the same spot as my last twinge? I go through the drill. I recall my conversation with Bob from across the street in Franklin. He beat pancreatic cancer fifteen-plus years ago. He still has twinges, he said, and when he does he attributes them to scar tissue. Relax, I tell myself. Scar tissue. But the twinge recurs. I shift positions, gently, hoping not to wake Burton because he sleeps too little as it is and there's no point in both of us losing sleep over my twinge. Still worried, I slip out of bed, slide my journal from the drawer of my nightstand and take it into the next room. I switch on a low light, flip to the first blank page and date the top. I write the word *Health* in the margin and describe my symptom. Unlike my husband, my journal is purely neutral, my detached but devoted nighttime friend. It doesn't frown or wince or urge me to call the doctor. It simply accepts what I say, witnesses my concern and gives me a bit of peace knowing I expressed my worry, that the next time I have a twinge my journal will remind me of the earlier one. And if that notation was a few days back, that twinge must have gone away or it would have come up again between the entry about the day Alexis and I ate plastic sandwiches and the time Camryn scribbled a picture for me.

I tiptoe back to bed and slip between the sheets, and then I remember the time I played golf with someone new in Florida. On the 12th tee of the West Course, she mentioned a friend who'd had a pain in his shoulder. He turned out to have bone cancer and died soon after. The story came on so fast that I didn't have time to broadcast my usual warning: I only want to hear good cancer stories. I took a chunk of grass on my drive. My heel had been sore for several days. Arthritis, I had assumed, an inconvenient result of aging. But hearing about bone cancer, I wondered. Two days later I called Dr. Malone. He answered my question without a note of exasperation, just the steady, matter-of-fact tone I appreciated about him. "Suzy, you do not have heel cancer." Within a couple of days, my heel stopped hurting.

By then, if I'm lucky, my mind has settled down and my twinge has subsided. Knowing your body once produced tumors is a humbling awareness. If it happened before, it could happen again.

The now is the sweet spot. When I gaze at a full moon in a clear sky or come up with the perfect word while writing on my laptop or behold the brazen yellow of a bed of daffodils on a springtime walk, when I hear the Canadian Tenors sing Leonard Cohen's "Hallelujah," when I taste a ripe peach or smell a leaf of fresh basil, I am fine and fearless in that instant. When I'm on the golf course, if I concentrate on my swing, if I turn, hinge, extend and finish, my golf ball occasionally makes a long, graceful arc and I stand in breathless joy admiring it. A well-executed golf shot results from hitting the ball on the sweet spot. It is a thing of beauty, and it only happens when I focus.

Staying in the moment is also a matter of focus. I will spend the rest of my hopefully long life working on it.

Should you be attending a lively dinner party, where the drinks and the conversation are flowing, there are two subjects best avoided. This story has been about both of them. In many circles, talking about cancer and talking about God are serious buzz killers. The first can be enough of a downer to destroy the flavor of duck cassoulet. The second topic, I have noticed, can arouse the same lack of enthusiasm. When I've told people the subject of my book, some have said, "I can't wait to read it." Others have said, "interesting," which is what we say when we don't want to say what we really think, polite code for, "I'm out of here." The great twentieth-century theologian Paul Tillich once said, "I hope for the day when everyone can speak again of God without embarrassment." That day has not yet arrived, which is why, dear reader, if you have stuck with me to this point, I am humbled and grateful.

Someone helping to usher in that day may be Tim Tebow. I've become a fan of the pro football player, a born-again Christian who publically expresses his religious sentiment. In college he wore biblical verses in the eye black under his eyes (not permitted in pro ball). As quarterback for the Denver Broncos, after scoring touchdowns, he knelt in prayerful thanks. In 2012, in an AFL wild-card game against the Pittsburgh Steelers, the Broncos were underdogs. On the first play of overtime, Tebow threw an 80-yard pass for a 29-23 win. Soon after, his game stats were announced. He had thrown 316 yards and set an NFL playoff record with 31.6 yards for completion. One of Tebow's favorite biblical verses is John 3:16. He wore the numbers penned beneath his eyes when he led the Florida Gators to victory in the 2009 college football National Championship game. God works in strange ways ... off the field and on.

Having a numerical miracle of my own, I did a little research on numerology. My personal favorite Godsign came to me through the oddly diverse sources of a gold bracelet and an aluminum license plate. In looking up the significance of number 26, I learned about correspondence tables. A correspondence table is a system in which an object or concept is linked by mystical connections according to an organizing principle. Numbers are a common organizing principle. Like the Hebrew alphabet, which first clued me in to the number 26, the English alphabet becomes a correspondence table when its letters are given numerical value. In the correspondence table for the English alphabet, A=1, B=2, etc., up to Z=26.

God has different names in many languages and faiths. Mohammed spoke of 99 names. Hindu scripture contains 1,000 names of Vishnu. Judaism, 72 names for El or Elohim. Sikhs refer to Waheguru or Nirankar; Hindus to Brahma or Krishna; Native Americans to Gitche Manitou; and, across the diverse continents of Asia and Africa, the divine spirit is invoked under dozens of names.

In English, we commonly use the simple, powerful word, God. What I read in my research on correspondence tables and the English language caused me to once again shake my head in wonder. I realized I had been given another clue to a mystery I would never fathom. The total of the numerical values in the word G-O-D: 26.

As the Duchess says to Alice in Wonderland, "Tut, tut, child! Everything's got a moral, if only you can find it."

On July 26, 2010, Burton and I enjoyed a date night up north at the farm. The day marked the sixth anniversary of my initial diagnosis. Each year away from the onset of cancer is an accomplishment. The more there are, the better the chance you might have beaten cancer for good. Puh, puh, puh!

We stayed home and shared drinks on the screened porch. It was one of those warm evenings I call primo porch nights. The summer had been full of such nights. There was a gentle breeze from the west. The Rose of Sharon tree just beyond our porch had begun to puff out with magenta blossoms the size of corsage carnations. A hummingbird darted back and forth between the flowers and the feeder which Burton kept filled with red nectar.

Burton arose from his rocking chair and walked over to the swing where I sat with my feet up. He clinked his chilled beer mug against my glass of pinot noir.

"To your special anniversary," he said.

"To the one who made it possible."

In the interest of truth, I should pause for a qualifier. As saintly as Burton's behavior was during those grueling months of my cancer experience, in recent years my co-survivor had reverted to being human. For instance, if I asked my husband where he was on a given day, he might bark that he'd already told me. If I dared interrupt when he was telling a long-winded story, he would growl or, worse yet, turn silent. He'd tell me he wanted to spend an evening with this or that couple and then complain when I booked too many dates. The typical Mars/Venus interactions that physically healthy couples are lucky enough to share. (Not, by the way, that I was so flawless.) But, on this particular night, Burton was mellowed by a couple of Fosters. I had his full attention.

Legs stretched out on the cushion, I swang from side to side. On the table in front of me, a paperback lay open. The book had been loaned to me by Ginger, my friend with the labyrinth. Undaunted by her MS, Ginger had undertaken a challenging Ph.D. program in depth psychology. She was studying mythological archetypes to understand the human psyche. I told Burton about what I was reading. My husband was often too distracted to hear me discuss abstract ideas, but this night, he listened.

"The ancients had an expression for the love of their story, whatever it was, however painful. They called it *amor fati*. With all the problems I've faced and lessons I've learned, my past made me who I am. It helped make our kids who they are, and our grandchildren. The story is mine. I love it for that."

"Artsy-fartsy whatever," Burton said. "We've both faced problems. We've both made mistakes. But we are who we are. I'm just glad we're still here together, sharing our porch."

"And sharing our stories."

We sat listening to the breeze and the birds and my creaking swing. Burton, like most men, tries to fix things. He walked into the house, returned with a can of WD-40 and sprayed it on the hinges of the swing. Now the swing not only creaked, it also smelled of oil. I thanked Burton for trying. Creaking, I realized, was part of the swing. If I wanted to take the ride, I had to put up with the creak.

We lingered on the porch savoring the balmy weather until 8:30 when we dragged ourselves into the house to make dinner. Burton sautéed perch from nearby John Cross Fisheries, where we had bought supremely fresh fish for over forty years. I had baked a sweet potato. I adored sweet potatoes; Burton didn't. He was stubborn about foods he didn't like, cooked peas for instance, and it was hard to sway him. Unless he was on one of his many diets, my husband's idea of potato consumption was Lays Potato Chips with a dip he concocted of cream cheese, ketchup and Tabasco. (Burton's attraction to the artery-clogging snack may have helped Detroit gain the dubious ranking of Potato Chip Consumption Capital of the World.)

That night I lobbied for sweet potatoes. "They're loaded with beta-Carotene, they don't need sour cream or butter, and they're naturally sweet," I said.

Burton wrinkled his nose doubtfully. "Okay, okay. I'll try."

I cut my sweet potato in half. Burton used his fork to deliver a morsel to his mouth, then lopped off a bigger bite. Soon he had consumed his half. I applied myself to my dinner, as though I didn't notice.

"Not bad," he said.

I considered Burton's willingness to eat a sweet potato a small victory for his nutritional health. "If this is out there, what else is out there?" I said. We had been quoting Naven R. Johnson for over twenty-five years. Sharing inside jokes and not needing to explain common references were among the joys of being together for so long, among the delicate but strong ties of marriage.

We rinsed the dishes together, and then Burton walked outside. Through the open window, he called, "Come here. Now."

I had not experienced many new Godsigns recently. I believed they were still out there, but I hadn't noticed them because I wasn't looking. It felt good to no longer fear my imminent demise on an hourly basis. I dried my hands and joined Burton where he stood in the gravel driveway.

Burton stretched his arm out, pointing to the east. "Look at that."

I looked past the old silo that still stood tall although the adjoining barn burned down in the sixties. I looked across the grassy field with the two-track that led to the lake. In the clear sky just above the serpentine line of treetops, a giant full moon arose. It was sweet-potato orange.

Goose bumps popped up on my skin.

"Hang on," Burton said. He strode to his truck and pulled out a pair of Swarovski crystal binoculars. Burton loves toys, whether they're viewfinders or the latest lob wedges for golf, ear protectors for shooting trap or skeet, or high-powered binoculars to check out deer in the fields. He looked through the binoculars, then handed them to me.

Through crystal lenses, the giant moon appeared even bigger. Wisps of cloud streaked across the eyes of the man in the moon. He looked to be wearing a blindfold, and then the clouds shifted and a mask covered his mouth. And then the clouds passed, and the moon was clear and brilliant once more. Godsigns are a lot like moons. When the sky is filled with clouds, the moon is invisible. But it is still there, whether we see it or not.

"A clear sky and a sweet-potato moon on my sixth anniversary," I said. "Now *that* is a Godsign." Then I hung the binoculars over my shoulder and took Burton's hands in mine. I pressed our clasped hands to my chest in a gesture of prayer.

Bowing my head, I repeated words I had voiced countless times over the past few years, words so many have voiced before: "*Baruch HaShem.*"

A Message for Co-Survivors

A BATTLE WITH ILLNESS is fought by many and shared with those you love. Here are some lessons I've learned from the front lines.

1. A patient needs an advocate. Listen with a level head. Ask tough questions. Keep track of the answers.
2. Be diligent. The first treatment regimen provides your best chance for beating cancer.
3. Get a second opinion.
4. Keep a list of others to call if the patient needs support. Have names and numbers of recent cancer survivors. We found help from Imerman Angels, which provides one-on-one support by linking patients with someone who faced a similar illness: or 312/274-5529.
5. Don't feel you have to "fix" a patient's attitude. Dispense hugs liberally.

6. Stay connected with friends.

7. Encourage your patient to seek spiritual support.

8. You may need support, too. If you need it, get it.

9. Create experiences for a patient to look forward to. (A yogurt smoothie, a walk, a visit from a friend or family member, a massage.)

10. Know the sun will shine again... eventually.

You are not alone. God bless.

Burton Farbman

Acknowledgments

I THANK BURTON Farbman, my rock and co-survivor, for championing my treatment, sharing in my saga and supporting my literary efforts. Anne Towbes, my auxiliary memory, conscience and best promoter. David Crumm, who helped to shape my story and overcame his reluctance to read about certain beleaguered parts of my anatomy. John Hile, Jane Wells, Celeste Dykas and Karen Campbell for helping me refine and promote my story. Rick Nease for also appreciating full moons.

I thank David and Nadine Farbman, Andy and Amy Farbman, Alexis, Camryn and Lindsay Farbman, Hunter, River and Fischer Farbman, my flesh and blood legacy and inspiration.

Thanks to Dr. Ira Mickelson, Lynn Sinclair Buehler, Barbara Loren Snyder and Ginger Winter for early reading and steady encouragement. To Denise Tietze for many years of superb back-up and to Tammy Nabozny for recent help. To Thelma Hardy and Rodney Lange for tech support. To John D. Lamb and Springfed Arts; Irina Reyn and Lizzie Skurnick for writing inspiration. To Earl Mackey and the C.G. Jung Society of Sarasota for improving my understanding of Jungian psychology.

Thanks to Anita, Arlene, Bobbye, Brenda, Cara, Danny, Denyse, Donna, Elaine, Jackie, Jill, Julie, Laurie, Lisa, Louie, Mary Lou, Mickey, Nancy, Natalie, Pat, Peggy, Rick, Rita, Sandi, Sandy, Shelley, Sue, Tonia, Zina, and so many other friends for never telling me I was crazy, even if I sometimes was.

Thanks to my sister LOCC 18 holers for putting up with my golf game when my time on the practice range was often supplanted by time at the keyboard.

And thanks to book club members and leaders everywhere whose joy in reading makes writers possible and all those solitary hours worthwhile.

About the Author

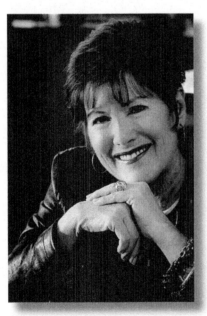

GODSIGNS IS SUZY Farbman's second memoir. She also wrote *Back from Betrayal, Saving a Marriage, a Family, a Life*. Prior to that, Suzy was a journalist for more than thirty years. She spent five years as a regional design editor for *Better Homes and Gardens* and other Meredith publications. She has been a contributing editor for *Detroit Monthly* magazine, concentrating on decorating, fashion and the arts; a columnist and feature writer for the *Detroit News*; a correspondent for *Women's Wear Daily*; and a freelance writer for national magazines including *Cosmopolitan*. She worked on public relations projects for the Farbman Group, as well. Profits from *Godsigns* will go to cancer research.

Suzy invites readers to share their own Godsigns with her and hopes to include their stories in her next book.

Suzy is available for book readings and speaking engagements. More information is available at www.GodsignsBook. com [http://www.GodsignsBook.com].

Contact Suzy at Godsigns@farbman.com

Colophon

READ THE SPIRIT Books produces its titles using innovative digital systems that serve the emerging wave of readers who want their books delivered in a wide range of formats—from traditional print to digital readers in many shapes and sizes. This book was produced using this entirely digital process that separates the core content of the book from details of final presentation, a process that increases the flexibility and accessibility of the book's text and images. At the same time, our system ensures a well-designed, easy-to-read experience on all reading platforms, built into the digital data file itself.

David Crumm Media has built a unique production workflow employing a number of XML (Extensible Markup Language) technologies. This workflow, allows us to create a single digital "book" data file that can be delivered quickly in all formats from traditionally bound print-on-paper to nearly any digital reader you care to choose, including Amazon Kindle®, Apple iBook®, Barnes and Noble Nook® and other devices that support the ePub and PDF digital book formats.

And due to the efficient "print-on-demand" process we use for printed books, we invite you to visit us online to learn more about opportunities to order quantities of this book with the possibility of personalizing a "group read" for your organization or congregation by putting your organizations logo and name on the cover of the copies you order. You can even add your own introductory pages to this book for your church or organization.

During production, we use Adobe InDesign®, <Oxygen/>® XML Editor and Microsoft Word® along with custom tools built in-house.

The print edition is set in Minion Pro and Myriad Pro.

Cover art and Design by Rick Nease: www.RickNeaseArt.com.

Editing by David Crumm.

Copy editing and XML styling by Celeste Dykas.

Digital encoding and print layout by John Hile.

If you enjoyed this book, you may also enjoy

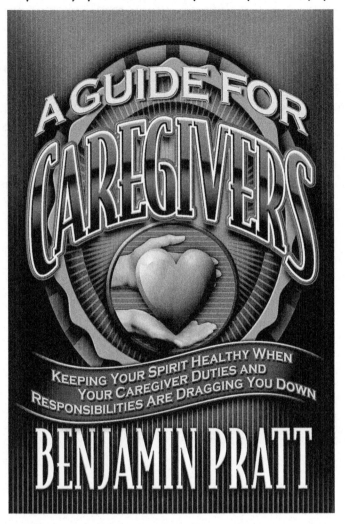

In one out of three households, someone is a caregiver: women and men who give of body, mind and soul to care for the well being of others. They need daily, practical help in reviving their spirits and avoiding burnout.

http://www.GuideForCaregivers.com

ISBN: 978-1-934879-27-6

If you enjoyed this book, you may also enjoy

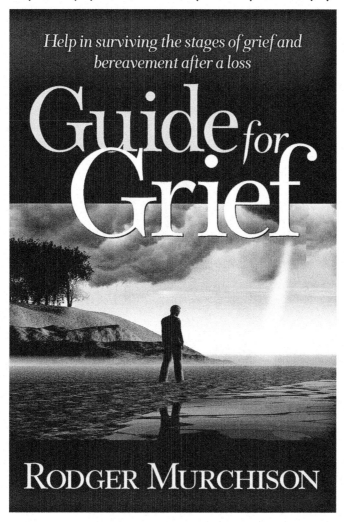

In his new Guide for Grief, the Rev. Rodger Murchison brings years of pastoral experience and study, sharing recommendations from both scripture and the latest research into loss and bereavement.

http://www.GuideForGrief.com

ISBN: 978-1-934879-31-3

If you enjoyed this book, you may also enjoy

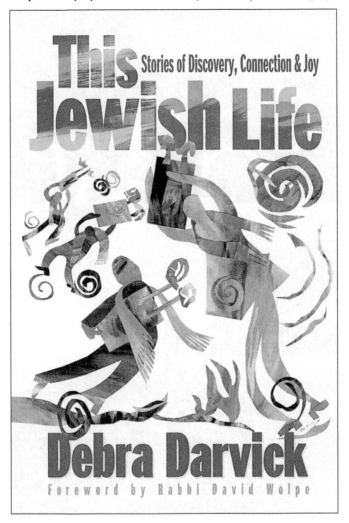

In "This Jewish Life: Stories of Discover, Connection, and Joy", fifty-five voices enable readers to experience a calendar's worth of Judaism's strengths—community, healing, transformation of the human spirit and the influence of the Divine.

http://www.ThisJewishLife.com

ISBN: 978-1-934879-36-8

If you enjoyed this book, you may also enjoy

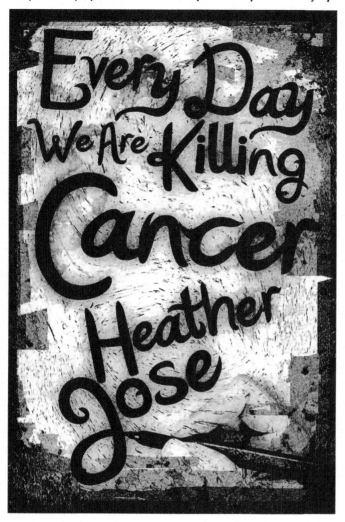

A hand-lettered sign, "We are killing cancer every day," traveled with the family on a long journey that ended in success. This is the story that is inspiring cancer thrivers nationwide.

http://www.EveryDayWeAreKillingCancer.com

ISBN: 978-1-934879-76-4

CPSIA information can be obtained
at www.ICGtesting.com
Printed in the USA
BVOW06*0955041217
501579BV00016B/24/P